About the Author

Pauline Wills is a qualified reflexologist, colour practitioner and yoga instructor. She is the founder member of the Oracle School of Colour where she teaches and runs a complementary therapy practice. She is the author of several books on reflexology, colour therapy and on the integration of both these therapies.

Colour Healing

Piatkus Guides

Other titles in this series include

A PIATKUS GUIDE

Colour Healing

Pauline Wills

PIATKUS

© 1999 Pauline Wills

First published in 1999 by
Judy Piatkus (Publishers) Ltd
5 Windmill Street, London W1P 1HF

The moral rights of the author have been asserted

A catalogue record for this book is available from the British Library

ISBN 0-7499-1933-7

Set in 12.5/14pt Perpetua
Typeset by Action Publishing Technology Limited, Gloucester
Printed & bound in Great Britain by
Mackays of Chatham PLC

Contents

Introduction

My awareness and love of colour developed many years ago when I was studying yoga. Practising yogic positions brought to me the realisation that by concentrating on the colours radiated by the chakras while working with specific postures, the energy flow of the chakra was increased. This realisation served to increase my love of and fascination for colour. I yearned to learn more.

By chance – if anything happens by chance – a friend told me of a colour healing course advertised at her local library. This course was being run by Lily Cornford, Principal of the Maitreya School of Colour Healing, and I enrolled. Through the knowledge imparted by this special woman, my under-standing of the vibrational energies of colour grew, culminating in my qualification as a colour practitioner.

After qualifying, Lily invited me to work with her, and this provided me with a unique opportunity to practise colour therapy. Under the strict discipline and ever watchful eye of Lily, I experienced and witnessed the power of colour as a healing energy, not just physically, but also mentally, emotionally and spiritually. I also came to understand that complete wellness requires all aspects of ourselves to be in a state of balance. Reflecting on this made me realise that the only person who can really heal is the person who has the disease. For most people, this is a hard concept to digest. We are all conditioned that our doctor takes care of our health and our only responsibility lies in, for example, remembering to take prescribed tablets three times a day. Unfortunately this is far from the case. I believe that the physical body is a mirror that reflects what is happening on all levels of our being. For example, if we are emotionally upset and are unable to resolve and work with the cause of these feelings, they will eventually manifest as a physical disease. Working with this concept made me realise that a complete cure can only happen if the initial cause is resolved. Striving to heal the physical symptom only can result in the cause manifesting a disease elsewhere in the body.

During the time that I have worked as a colour practitioner, I have frequently found that a person is aware of the cause of their illness but finds this explanation too painful or difficult to work with. My belief is that all illness gives us a chance to look at ourselves and to change those things to which we no longer resonate. Doing this will ultimately result in a heightening of our vibrational frequency and progression along life's evolutionary spiral. I know through my own experiences that no change comes without discomforts, but the benefits arising from the change far outweigh them. Unfortunately we only realise this when the change has been made and we are walking along our new chosen path. I feel that it is important to remember that we have been given the free will either to allow changes to take place or to remain, for the time being, where we stand at present.

As well as teaching yoga and working as a colour practitioner, I also work as a qualified reflexologist. While travelling with a colleague to help run a colour therapy course, I intuitively realised that I had to combine colour with reflexology and gradually, over the following two years, information was channelled through me on how this was to be done. As I worked with these new techniques, I saw how the combination of the two therapies amplified the healing process and worked with ailments difficult to treat with reflexology alone. Colour also proved to be a tremendous boon to people suffering painful feet because it removed the stagnated energy, the cause of the discomfort, painlessly. Further proof of this was given when I was invited to work in palliative care as a complementary practitioner as terminally ill patients often experience pain in their feet and find the pressure techniques of reflexology extremely uncomfortable. Using colour achieves the same results, without the pain. These patients also taught me that colour aids relaxation, reduces the feeling of nausea often caused by drugs and aids in the relief of constipation induced by morphine. All of this ultimately helped these people to die with dignity. This, I feel, is extremely important.

As my sensitivity to colour increased, I became very aware of how the colours I wore and with which I was surrounded affected me. I found myself needing to wear one colour during the morning and a different one later in the day. This need for a variety of different coloured clothes proved to be a problem, because the colours of clothes are dictated by the fashion industry. If the shade that you require is not in season then the chances of acquiring it are practically nil. The way that I overcame this was to wear different coloured scarves. I also visited local Indian dress shops and found many exciting items of clothing in the most exquisitely coloured materials. Another discovery that I made during this time was connected with the colours in my home, which would please and resonate with me one day, but dismay me on others. This proved a problem, because it is neither practical nor financially viable to constantly refurbish and redecorate one's home. I overcame this by painting the walls white and introducing colour in furnishings and fittings. If these are kept simple, they are not too expensive to change as the need arises.

Nature was another source of colour that nurtured me with its energies. Walking in the country or being in the garden, among the variegated seasonal flowers, induced in me a wonderful sense of peace and relaxation. I learned to feel the vibrant colours displayed by trees and plants and to absorb the earth's energies by walking bare-foot on the grass. I also found great joy in the colours reflected in crystals and stones. I found their differing energies both stimulating and healing. I started to collect crystals and in time knew which crystal I needed to work with at any given time. All of these experiences have taught me to respect nature as a living entity.

After working as a complementary practitioner for some time, I felt the need to share with others the knowledge that had been imparted to me. I embarked upon this by running introductory days on the vibrational energies of colour and giving talks to small groups of people. This led me to devise and teach a certified course for qualified reflexologists who wished to integrate colour with reflexology, and finally to starting the Oracle School of Colour. The contact with and feedback from the students who pass through the school have given me great insight into myself, alongside increasing my own knowledge through the many ways I have had to invent to help these students understand the basic principles of colour healing. For this I thank those who have already qualified and those who are still in the process. Teaching to me is a great and enjoyable challenge and an even greater learning experience. I hope that I will be given the privilege to continue for many more years.

One aim of this book is to inspire you to understand colour with its many shades and hues and the powers that colour and light have to affect us on a physical, emotional, mental and spiritual level. When discussing colour healing one frequently encounters sceptics who dismiss it before they have heard the explanations. I recommend that they read about colour and work positively with it before dismissing it as merely something that gives either pleasure or displeasure to the eye. Disbelieving the effectiveness of anything conditions our bodies to reject it, as shown in both complementary and allopathic medicine. If colour therapy is used with animals, outstanding results can be achieved, because they automatically accept it without question. I have seen this with my own cats, one in particular. She was very sick with a high temperature because of a viral infection. She lay on her side, refusing all food and drink and appearing very sorry for herself. If I tried to give her water through a tiny dropper, she would bring it back up. I started to treat her twice a day, with both coloured light and using colour with contact healing. After each treatment she showed improvement and actually started to purr when the coloured light was focused on her. Within a remarkably short time she made a complete recovery.

In allopathic medicine, the role of our mind in the effectiveness of treatment has also been shown. Placebo pills have been given to terminally ill people who have been told that they are receiving a new wonder drug that has proven to be greatly beneficial for the disease they are suffering. After taking the placebo for a time their health starts to improve, but as soon as they learn the true nature of the tablets they relapse. This has taught me never to underestimate the power of the mind and its effect upon the physical body. If we are able to think positively about the healing power of colour, we will gain positive results. If we think negatively, we block its energy and very little transpires.

A further aim of this book is to give you some insight into the healing role of colour, to share ways that will help you to grow in colour awareness and to describe techniques that you can use to enhance your own state of well-being. I would suggest that you first read through the book to gain an overall picture of colour before starting to work with any of the exercises, so that you can discover the techniques that you think will work for you. When we enjoy doing something, an element of fun is brought into the exercise, enhancing the results. Starting in this way encourages us to look at those aspects of colour that we at first considered boring or uninteresting to find out how they are able to help us.

The book shows that there are several ways of working with colour. One way is with a bag of coloured ribbons, explained in Chapter 4. When you have selected a ribbon from the bag, look up its colour attributes, then work with the colour using any of the techniques described in later chapters. You could breathe in the colour with one of the breathing techniques, or work with visualisation or with one of the mandalas, making your chosen colour the dominant one among any others you choose to work with. You could also wear a scarf or item of clothing in this colour for the rest of the day.

If you intuitively know the colour that would be most beneficial for you, there is no need to select one from your bag of coloured ribbons. Simply choose from the book a way of working with the colour you need. Continue to work with this colour until you feel attracted to a different colour. If we are drawn towards a colour it usually indicates that at some level we need it. When it no longer attracts us, we no longer need it.

If you are suffering from a specific complaint, such as depression or anxiety, the chapter on visualisation illustrates ways of helping yourself to overcome this. As well as working with the suggested visualisation technique, it is important to try to find the cause of your condition and the best way to resolve it. Colour may temporarily relieve the symptoms, but if the cause is not worked with, the symptoms will return.

The final chapter examines some of the ways in which colour is professionally used in therapy. It also gives a list of the colours most beneficial for relieving simple ailments and describes ways for working with them. What is very important to remember is the need to consult your own doctor for his or her advice if you suffer any physical disease. Never replace with colour any treatment that you have been prescribed. The only person who should instruct you to stop taking medication is the person who has prescribed it, and that is your doctor. Being on prescribed drugs does not prevent you from working with colour; in fact it is something to be recommended, because it will help the healing process and give you a greater sense of well-being.

When working with colour you should not use coloured light unless you are a qualified colour practitioner. Some coloured lights can have contra-indications and, unless you know what these are, the exercise becomes detrimental instead of beneficial. An extreme example of this is the use of strobe lighting in nightclubs. This has been shown to trigger epileptic fits and aggression in young people. Another example is the use of red light on a person suffering high blood pressure. Instead of helping the condition, red light aggravates it.

I hope that you enjoy working with the book and benefit from the exercises. What is important is to remember that to achieve any results, practice on a regular basis is essential, requiring both discipline and time. But I am sure that you will feel the effort worthwhile once you start to experience the wonderful benefits of colour. Although it is many years since I started on my journey, I am aware that there is still a great deal for me to learn and to experience before my life ends.

1

What is Colour
Healing?

Be thou the rainbow to the storms of life

Byron

How many of you have experienced a sense of joy and
wonder when looking at a glorious sunset, felt depressed on
a grey, cloudy day, or experienced a sense of peace and
relaxation upon entering a room decorated in the pastel
shades of blue, green or violet. These feelings are your reac-
tion to the colours' vibrational energies. Your aura, the
electromagnetic field that surrounds all living things, also
reflects how you are feeling and the state of your physical
health through the colours it displays. This is expressed in
well-known sayings: 'I feel blue today'; 'She looks green
with envy'; 'He is in a black mood.' I believe that these
expressions developed at a time when more people were
gifted enough to see the aura, because if one is depressed the
aura reflects a dark dingy blue, if envious it turns a muddy
shade of green and if we are in a foul mood many of the
colours are missing, leaving black patches throughout the

auric field. All dull, dark shades reflect the negative aspects of a colour, while bright clear shades show the positive ones.

Colour affects us because it is an energy that is capable of altering our biochemical structure. The energy that emanates from the sun and is seen by us as light has different vibrational energies that we see as the colours of nature, as observed in rainbows in the sky after storms. Early man must have wondered at this phenomenon and questioned why the colours always appeared in the same order. Not until 1665 was the mystery solved, when Isaac Newton, a young student of physics, was working in his laboratory. He noticed that a shaft of light entering the room through a small aperture passed through a prism lying on his desk. Out of the opposite side of the prism appeared the colour spectrum, leading him to deduce that white light must contain the colours of the spectrum. To prove his theory, he placed a second inverted prism approximately six inches from the first. When the spectral colours produced from the first prism passed through the second one, they re-emerged as white light. Newton then went on to show that this occurred because the prism refracted light; as each colour has a different angle of refraction, the colours appeared separately and always in the same order.

The living energy of the vibrational frequencies of these spectral colours is used in colour healing, alongside the healing power of light from the sun.

The History of Colour Healing

Colour is a very ancient form of holistic treatment. In his books on the 'lost civilisation' of Atlantis, Frank Alpers describes circular healing temples with domed roofs constructed from interlocking crystals which refracted the light as it passed through them, flooding the temple with the spectral colours. Around the circumference of the temple he suggests that the Atlanteans built individual healing rooms fitted with crystal doors that could be energised to the frequency of the colour required. These rooms were not used solely for treating disease but also for healing relation-ships, for childbirth and in assisting the transition of the soul from this life to the next.

According to the findings of archaeologists, healing temples built by early Egyptian civilisations were lavishly decorated and also had healing rooms constructed within them. Those attending for healing were colour diagnosed before being placed into the room radiating the prescribed colour. Alongside this form of treatment, herbs, salves, dyes and coloured minerals were also used. The minerals were usually worn in the belief that they supplied a continuous flow of the colour's energy. The Egyptians also believed that the wearing of bracelets or rings stopped the loss of energy and prevented them from picking up any negative energy.

In India, a country naturally alive with colour, minerals and gemstones were employed to provide the colour frequencies needed to promote healing, in the belief that these were a concentration of the seven cosmic rays. They would either be boiled for several hours in water that would then be diluted to homeopathic potencies for patients to drink, or be burned so that the ash could be used medici-nally. The use of precious as well as semi-precious gems made this a very costly treatment. To give healing in absentia gem ash was placed on a rotating wheel, at the centre of which was placed an image of the person requesting healing. It was believed that the rotating gem ash released its frequency to the person in the image.

The ancient Greeks were noted for their healing practices.

The city of Heliopolis was famous for its healing temples, which were designed to refract sunlight in a similar way to both the Atlantean and Egyptian temples. Many of the forefathers of modern medicine originated here, including Hippocrates, a physician born on the island of Cos who is believed to have followed the Greek healing system, which explained the mechanism of illness in terms of the four basic humours or bodily fluids. The blood (red) was connected to the heart, yellow bile was associated with the spleen, black bile arose in the brain and phlegm (white) was identified with the liver. It has been suggested that Hippocrates was an alchemist and as such employed both colour and magic in his healing techniques. To produce colour he would have worked with flowers, coloured plasters, ointments and minerals.

With the advent of the Christian era, the medical practices of colour were deemed pagan and banned, driving it underground. Most of the written material containing the ancient wisdom of colour therapy was lost. Whatever has survived was passed on by word of mouth. It was not until the 7th century that colour therapy was revived by Avicenna, a Persian. He was reputed to be a child prodigy and during his lifetime wrote approximately 100 books. The most renowned of these was *The Canon*, in which he made reference to his own ideas and findings on the use of colour for diagnosis and in treatment, including his observations of the adverse effects that colour can produce. He appears to have used mainly the primary colours red, blue and yellow. Red, he noted, increased blood pressure, while blue lowered it. Yellow, he proclaimed, reduced inflammation and pain. For his coloured brews, he used flowers and sunlight.

During the Renaissance, an outstanding healer who incorporated colour into his treatments was Theophrastus Bombastus von Hohenheim, known as Paracelsus. Paracelsus was born near Zurich, held a doctor's degree and developed great interest in alchemy, astrology and the occult sciences. His medical outlook was holistic, acknowledging the Chinese system of working with the elements of earth, water, fire and air alongside the physical, astral, mental and spiritual aspects of a person. His interest in alchemy led to him using herbs, minerals and coloured light in his medical practice.

The early 19th century saw great advances in medicine that overshadowed the use of colour therapy until 1877, when Dr Seth Pancoast, from Philadelphia, published a book entitled *Blue and Red Lights*, in which he explained his form of treatment using these two colours. He believed that the red ray accelerated the nervous system and the blue light relaxed it. To administer these colours he used glass filters. A year later, Dr Edwin Babbitt, from Hamden, New York, published *The Principles of Light and Colour*, which explained his understanding of the spectral colours and their effectiveness in treating disease. To administer colour he invented a cabinet called the Thermoline, which made use of natural daylight. He later remodelled it to incorporate a chromodisc, to which he fitted coloured filters and an electric arc, which provided the source of light. His treatments included water solarised with colour for his patients to drink.

Not until the early part of the 20th century did colour come to the forefront as a therapy, mainly because of the work of Rudolph Steiner, a Hungarian from Kraljevec, and Dinshah P. Ghadiali who worked in Malaga, New Jersey. Steiner was regarded as an occultist, philosopher, teacher and religious leader, and he predicted that colour would play a very important part in medicine during the 21st century. He believed that illness was caused by the separation of earthly consciousness from higher perception and that the best way of reuniting these two aspects of ourselves was through art. The colours he used were red, blue, yellow, green, white, black and peach blossom, which he divided into two categories. He called red, blue and yellow the image colours and he related white, black, green and peach blossom to mathematical form, believing that form had the power to amplify the healing effect of colour. His work is still being taught in the Rudolph Steiner schools that he founded.

In 1934 Dinshah Ghadiali published his three-volume work, the *Spectro-Chrome Metry Encyclopedia*, which constituted a home training course. Ghadiali was well versed in electricity, mathematics and physics and, with his scientific background, he set out to formulate a scientific approach for the application of colour to the physical body. He worked with a twelve-colour system and invented two machines that transmitted the colours through slides. The first machine he called the Graduate Spectro-Chrome, which had revolving coloured slides housed in an aluminium slide carrier built into it. The second machine, called the Aluminium Spectro-Chrome, was smaller and intended for home use. Although Ghadiali had no medical training he was awarded four honorary medical degrees for his research into colour. When Ghadiali died in 1966, his son Darius assumed the presidency of the Spectrum Research Institute, which his father founded in Malaga in the United States. Because of continuing restrictions by the government against the Institute, he dissolved it and formed a non-profit, educational corporation named the Dinshah Health Society to continue the expansion of Spectro-Chrome knowledge.

Alongside Darius, other pioneers researched the field of colour therapy, experimenting with varying techniques of applications. Some of these pioneers have scientifically documented their results, others have not, but what is being shown is the powerful healing force of colours' vibrational energies, leading to more people finding out how colour can help them.

Colour Healing and Other Complementary Therapies

During the 1980s some complementary practitioners discovered that using the vibrational energies of colour with their own particular therapy enhanced the treatment, though some opposed this practice, believing that a therapy should be kept 'pure'. I personally believe that whatever therapy or combination of therapies helps a person is right for them.

In the United States, colour was recently introduced into acupuncture and given the name colourpuncture. This technique was founded and developed by Peter Mandel and involves administering the correct colour, in the form of light, to the acupuncture points. He found that by focusing coloured light on acupuncture points on the skin, powerful impulses were triggered in the physical and energy bodies. Colourpuncture is now available in the United Kingdom.

Another therapy to incorporate colour is Reiki, an ancient system of Japanese healing rediscovered in the late 19th century by Dr Mikao Usui, a Japanese scholar and monk. Reiki works with the universal lifeforce present in all things, which is activated and channelled through the hands of the practitioner when they make contact with the recipient. Colour is incorporated into this therapy through the visualisation of the required colour infusing the lifeforce. This technique is still in its infancy, so its effectiveness has not yet been fully ascertained.

A method of distance healing incorporating colour is radionics. Radionics was developed by Albert Abrahams of

San Francisco and is based on the theory that man together with all living forms is bathed in the electromagnetic field of the earth as well as being surrounded by its own energy field, the aura. If this vibrates to the wrong frequency, he maintains that disease will occur. In radionic therapy, the particular vibrations of each organ, disease and remedies are given in numerical values known as 'rates', which are transmitted via a radionics machine to a patient in order to promote healing. Recognising that each colour has its own vibrational frequency, the rates for this were found and transmitted in the same way. Another way of transmitting colour radionically was discovered in 1991 by Ryszard Olszack. Through radionics, he discovered a pattern that generates an energy called neo-energy, or the energy of shape. This, he found, produced all the colours of the spectrum and could restore any that were missing in a person's aura. He called his invention the PIMAT, or pyramid mat.

Colour can also be used in yoga. Apart from awakening and moving energy, the postures of yoga therapeutically affect the physical body. Both the movement of energy and therapeutic benefits are enhanced when colour is used. Each of the classical postures, when positioned correctly, works with one of the seven major chakras that support our endocrine system. Each chakra radiates one of the spectral colours; by visualising this colour filling and radiating out from the chakra into the aura while the posture is being held, it energises the body and brings the associated endocrine gland to balance. You will find more information on this in Chapter 5.

A number of complementary practitioners work with the Bach Flower Remedies alongside their chosen therapy. These remedies were originated by Dr Edward Bach, who in addition to orthodox medicine, practised homeopathy, believing that natural cures exist for every ailment. After suffering a severe illness he found that he could intuitively judge the healing properties of different plants and the illnesses they can cure. This led him to give up his Harley Street practice and settle in Wales, where he continued his search for healing plants. Because of the demand for treatment with these plants he devised a way of extracting and bottling their essence, which he then gave to his patients. This production method is still used today. The flower remedies are designed to treat the whole person, not just symptoms of illness. The principle behind their use is that every disorder, physical or psychological, arises because of an inner imbalance. In 1989, Ingrid S. Kraaz and Wulfing von Rohr added colour to these remedies with affirmations, meditations and visualisations. They believed the vibrational energy of the flower essences could be empowered with the vibrational energy of colour. When researching this, their observations showed positive effects on a person's well-being, which promoted their physical health. As a result of their work they devised the Original Bach Flower Color Card Set.

The therapy that I integrated with colour is reflexology, which teaches that the feet and hands are a mirror image of the entire physical body, with the left foot or hand representing the left side of the body and the right foot or hand representing the right side of the body. The feet and hands are divided into what are called 'reflexes' and each separate reflex is connected to an organ, muscle or bone. It is believed that the body contains energy channels through which lifeforce flows; if these become blocked with stagnated energy, disease can arise in the physical body. This stagnated energy, found through the presence of pain in the reflexes when massaged, can be dispersed with specific massage techniques. During many years practising reflexology I found certain people intolerant of the pain and therefore reluctant to continue treatment, even though they found it to be beneficial. Through research, I found the application of colour to the painful reflexes painlessly cleared the stagnated energy and helped the person to find and work with the cause of the disease. The application of colour with reflexology is described in Chapter 9.

I have learned about the research and successful use of colour in healing by former and present pioneers in this field observing many wonderful results. It leaves me in no doubt about colour's therapeutic power – mental, emotional, physical and spiritual.

2

Light

We are beings of light, therefore light is essential for our
well-being.

Sunlight, containing the vibrational frequencies of colour, is
vital for our well-being and has been used in healing throughout the ages. When we spend time outdoors, alongside
colour we absorb another very important ray, ultra-violet
light. The most beneficial way for the body to absorb both
colour and ultra-violet light is through eyes that are free from
spectacles or contact lenses because, as the experiments of
pioneers working with light proved, only a very small
percentage of ultra-violet light can pass through glass. This
does not mean that we have to spend long hours sitting in the
sun, which could be detrimental because overexposure of the
skin to ultra-violet light can cause skin cancer. What is beneficial is sitting or walking in the shade for at least half an hour
each day. Unfortunately modern life-styles frequently
prevent us from spending time outdoors. We tend to
commute by car, work in an office under artificial light,
return home by car and then spend what is left of the day in

front of the television. Along with other people working in this field, I feel that the general deprivation of light suffered by a large percentage of the population could be the cause of many diseases.

Light and Health

John Ott, a time-lapse photographer and pioneer in this field who has worked on many projects during his lifetime, was given an assignment to observe the growth of corn with time-lapse photography. He started by growing the corn in a greenhouse, but found that it was spindly. He also tried growing the corn outdoors, encasing it in a makeshift plastic enclosure when it reached a certain stage of development, and found that the corn now grew normally. This discovery led him to experiment with other plants in the same way; again, the result was that the plants growing under plastic sheeting were much healthier. What he ultimately learned from these experiments was that plastic allows up to 95 per cent of ultra-violet light to pass through, whereas most glass filters cut out 97 per cent of ultra-violet light. Because his plants and corn produced healthier growth under plastic he deduced that ultra-violet light was essential to their growth. This led him to consider whether or not the same principle applied to human beings.

John Ott suffered from an arthritic hip and was forced to move around with the aid of a cane. Medically he was advised that he would eventually need a hip replacement. Fortunately for him, he broke his glasses and was forced for a time to carry on his work without them. To his amazement, his hip started to improve, enabling him to dispose of his walking cane, to climb stairs and to play golf, things he had been unable to do for some time. He suspected that this was because of the ultra-violet light he was now able to absorb through his eyes. He therefore continued to work outdoors without glasses, with the result that his hip improved to the point where surgery was no longer necessary. His own improvement in health convinced him that ultra-violet light was as essential for humans as for plants.

The ability of ultra-violet light to pass through plastic lenses depends on the type of plastic used to make them. If you wear glasses and are interested in finding out more about your lenses ask your eye specialist for further information.

Dr Jane Wright, in charge of cancer research at Bellevue Medical Center in New York City, learned of John Ott's work and during the summer of 1959 agreed to instruct 15 of her patients to spend as much time as possible outdoors, without their glasses. Although the results were inconclusive, she did find that the cancer in 14 of the patients had not progressed and they reported feeling much better. The 15th patient reported that she felt no benefit from the exercise and tests showed that her tumour had grown in size. It was later discovered that she had misheard the instructions and had failed to remove her glasses.

Light entering the eyes aids the healthy functioning of the physical body by having a direct influence on the hypothalamus. This is shown in the work of another pioneer, Dr Jacob Liberman, a doctor of optometry. He also recognised the fact that exposure to sunlight influences a person both physiologically and psychologically, and in his book *Light Medicine of the Future* (1991), he emphasises that light is not important for vision alone but for the healthy functioning of the human body.

The hypothalamus serves as our biological clock, controlling the nervous system and stimulating our hormonal system through the light information it sends to the pineal gland. It also aids the production of vitamin D and calcium.

It is therefore believed that the metabolism of a living cell could be connected with the utilisation of the nutritional factors supplied by the energy of light.

Another disorder that has been recognised as being caused through light deprivation is seasonal affective disorder (SAD). This condition starts with the onset of autumn and disappears at the beginning of spring and its symptoms are lethargy, depression and a craving for carbohydrates. The cause is the lack of light available to the pineal gland during the short grey days of winter. One of the hormones secreted by this gland is melatonin, which I always think of as the hibernatory hormone. When the sun sets and darkness falls, the secretion of melatonin increases, telling us that it is time to sleep. With the onset of dawn, these secretions are greatly reduced, summoning the body to rise for the start of a new day. People suffering SAD have been shown to have high levels of melatonin in their bloodstream during daylight hours. This condition can now be remedied with the aid of a SAD light unit emitting full spectrum light, which a person is subjected to each day for a set length of time that depends upon the strength of the light unit.

Seasonal affective disorder is not the only condition to be helped by sunlight. A great deal of information is available about post-menopausal women suffering from osteoporosis, a condition of brittle bones caused by the loss of bony tissue. The decline in the levels of oestrogen and progesterone has been partially blamed for this. What is interesting is the news that this disease is now affecting quite a large percentage of men. Could this again result from our modern life-style, which separates us from the natural daylight that is so essential for the calcium production in our body?

A student attending an introductory workshop on the vibrational energies of colour reported that some months back she had undergone a bone scan that confirmed that she was suffering from osteoporosis. Her life-style was such that she had spent very little time outdoors. After receiving the hospital report, she made sure that she spent at least one hour a day in the open air. If the weather was warm and sunny, she sat in the garden; if not, she went for a walk. After six months had elapsed she returned to the hospital for a further bone scan and, to the amazement of the doctors, it showed a significant improvement in her bone density. She reported that now she never misses her 'daily dose of light'.

EXERCISE: WORKING WITH SUNLIGHT

It is preferable to practise this exercise in a secluded, shady place, outdoors.

☆ Sitting with your eyes open, visualise shafts of sunlight entering your eyes. Imagine your eyes to be an extension of your brain and as the light enters them feel the whole of your brain being illuminated. With each inhalation take the light down your spine to energise your spinal cord and the nerves that branch off from here to all the organs and muscles of your physical body. As your body starts to glow with light, feel the energy that it is generating.

☆ Bring your awareness back to your brain and your hypothalamus, which forms part of the forebrain – in the centre below the thalamus and above the pituitary gland – and is responsible for the metabolism of fat, carbohydrates and the water content of the body. It also regulates our body temperature and sleep patterns. See the hypothalamus glowing with the light that keeps all these functions operating smoothly.

☆ Finally, think about the ultra-violet rays contained in sunlight. These are not visible to the human eye, but you might like to visualise them as a dark translucent violet. Imagine these rays flowing from your brain, into your neck and interacting with your parathyroid glands to aid their metabolism of calcium and phosphorus to help with any skeletal problems you may be suffering. Now close your eyes for a short while and feel all of your body vibrating with its vital nutrient, light.

To gain any benefits from the exercises given in this book, they must be practised on a regular basis. You might find it helpful to keep a diary to record the benefits and difficulties that you experience. It can be very interesting occasionally to look back at what you have written. You can gain great insight into your progress.

Light and the Spirit

All life inhabiting the earth needs sunlight for survival. Without this, the earth would be an extinct planet. As human beings, we accept the sun's light because we are able to see by it and experience its many benefits, especially during the spring and summer months. What is not so tangible is our own spiritual light, the part of us that is eternal and originates from the Supreme Being. This light plays a role in various religions and esoteric paths, but to realise it within ourselves and to become integrated with it requires much inward searching, coupled with discipline. One of the ways to access our spiritual light is through the chakras and their colours (explained in Chapter 3). Each of the seven major chakras are rungs on the ladder leading to the Divine Light of consciousness. If we work with each chakra's colour and properties, our spiritual growth and understanding prospers.

From ancient civilisations to the present day, many religions and cultures have regarded colour as a manifestation of the light and for this reason ascribed it to deities and used it in religious rites. One reason for stained glass being used in Christian churches was the hope that the light the windows radiated would help man to remember his own inner light, which came from the Supreme Being. In Catholicism, at Easter the paschal candle is lit at the beginning of the rites for Holy Saturday to represent the light of the risen Christ as it is taken in procession through the church. I have heard it said that the many faces forming the Supreme Being are recognised by the colours radiating from them.

Many paths teach that the whole of creation came into force from the primordial light that emanated from the Supreme Being. Its action gave us two aspects of light. The androgynous Supreme Being brought forth its feminine aspect, which was spiritual light, and transformed this into the physical light of creation. Through this the whole of creation became imbued with that original spiritual light and it is this which forms the divine aspect of ourselves. In his book, *Light*, Omraam Mikhaël Aïvanhov, explains this event by saying that before God created, He called forth his feminine principle, which encompassed Him in a circle of light, the limits of which became the limits of the universe. Then, through the masculine principle, God projected into this light images, which crystallised and took on material form.

In esoteric literature and the Bible we frequently read that we, as human beings, are made in the image of God. If we believe this, it must mean that we also contain within ourselves both the creative and intuitive feminine principle and the intellectual masculine energy that is the intelligence behind that creative principle, and that we are encircled by an aura of light. It must also mean that our thoughts create forms that affect us, the environment and any person associated with that original thought. Being aware of this should make us more mindful of what we are thinking and endeavour to change any negative thoughts into positive ones. It should also encourage us to send thoughts of unconditional love to our fellow human beings, instead of thoughts that could prove to be destructive.

In order to become integrated with the Divine Light once more, we have to work towards wholeness. This entails integrating the feminine and masculine aspects of ourselves as we work with our body, mind and spirit. When we have been able to achieve this – and it can take many lifetimes – we reach the state of enlightenment, where we become one with the light of the Creator.

EXERCISE: WORKING WITH THE LIGHT

☆ Find a place that is quiet and warm, where you will not be disturbed. Sit down in a comfortable position, making sure that your spine is straight. Gently close your eyes and bring your concentration into your breath. With each exhalation, breathe out any tension in your physical body.

☆ When your body feels relaxed, bring your concentration to the crown of your head. Here you will see a narrow beam of white light, coming from the universe, entering your head. This beam of light is always present; it is our connection to the spirit world. As you concentrate on this light, imagine it increasing in size until it becomes the same diameter as the top of your head. When it has reached this dimension, picture it travelling through your body, completely filling it with light. Allow this light to work with any tension, pain or disease present and to re-energise all aspects of your being.

☆ On your next exhalation, envisage this light flowing out through the pores of your skin into the electromagnetic field of your aura that surrounds you. Continue to do this until you have built a bright circle of light around your physical body. Now sit quietly for a few moments, feeling the presence of this light and noting your experiences.

☆ Finally, consider your own spiritual light. What meaning has this for you? I believe that if we are to reach ultimate health, we have to become whole, and this means integrating our body, mind and spirit, which entails working with this light.

☆ When you are ready, start to increase your inhalation and exhalation and open your eyes.

3

The Aura: Our Coat
of Many Colours

Your aura is the key to your real self. It is the visible
expression of your mind, soul and spirit. Upon the
condition of your aura depends whether you are
experiencing the light within.

S.G.J. Ousley

Our aura is the electromagnetic field surrounding us, filled
with the constantly changing colours derived from light. The
vibrational energies of these colours integrate with the physical body to keep it healthy when they are in balance or to
manifest as disease when they are out of balance. An understanding of the aura and the colours it radiates is important
when working therapeutically with colour.

Although the majority of people are as yet unable to see
the aura, its living energy is very much a part of our being in
that it contains the emotional, mental and spiritual aspects of
our self. How we feel emotionally, think mentally and evolve
spiritually are portrayed by the colours present in the layers
of the aura linked to these parts of us. The physical body,

which is the visible part of the aura, to me represents the mirror that reflects our metaphysical state. If we are emotionally upset, mentally tired and harassed, the physical body will reflect this. Our spiritual awakeness (or otherwise) can be seen through our physical eyes. Our posture and speech can reveal blocked emotional or mental energies that need to be released if we are to flow with and absorb the ever abundant energy of life. When we allow ourselves to flow with this energy and learn to listen to and follow our intuition and discover and work with our spirituality, then our inner light starts to grow, displaying its presence by the colours present in our aura and felt through our physical sense of peace and well-being. For this to happen, we need to take time to look at and feel into ourselves. Part of this process is acknowledging and learning about the aura and the vibrational energies of its colours.

The Composition of the Aura

The aura consists of seven sheaths or layers, the first of these constituting the physical body. The remaining six layers interpenetrate with the physical body and each other. They can be likened to a set of Russian dolls that fit snugly inside each other because each doll is slightly larger. Likewise, each layer of the aura is slightly larger than its neighbour and therefore protrudes beyond it.

The aura is a vital and living part of us, expanding and contracting in accordance with our state of well-being. The full extent of its expansion depends on our spiritual awareness. It is reported that the aura of the Buddha extended for three miles. I am sure that this is also true for other enlightened beings such as the Christ.

The layers constituting the aura are filled with many

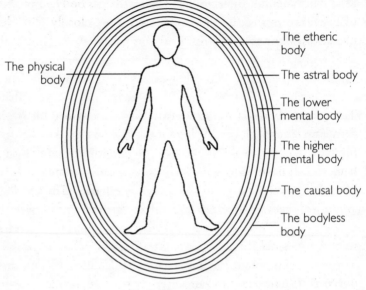

The etheric body

The astral body

The lower mental body

The higher mental body

The causal body

The bodyless body

The physical body

The aura

vibrant, flowing, ever changing colours and their vibrational energies. The colours displayed in the outer part of the aura are ethereal compared with the dense colours seen closer to the physical body. The colours present at any given moment are a reflection of our emotional, mental and spiritual state at that time. Bright, clear colours show a positive nature, whereas dark and dingy colours reveal negative attributes. If a person becomes very angry, the layer of the aura linked to our feelings becomes clouded with a dark dingy red, while envy produces a dull, dark green. These colours then infiltrate the other auric layers, finally manifesting as a physical 'feeling' that will eventually lead to disease if not dealt with. Disease that starts in the aura can be detected by locating areas that are either devoid of colour or vibrating to the wrong colour.

The layers that constitute the 'invisible' part of the aura are the etheric, the emotional (or astral), the lower mental, the higher mental, the causal and the bodyless body. The first of these layers and the one connected most closely with the physical body is the etheric.

The Etheric Body

The etheric body is the blueprint for our physical body. It forms the second layer of the aura and holds the key to our physical shape, size and gender, to the colour of our skin and hair. If we have an organ or limb surgically removed, the blueprint for it is still present in the etheric. This is why amputees report that they can still feel the missing limb.

The etheric body is filled with energy channels called nadis that work with the nervous system in the physical body. Through these channels flows prana, or lifeforce. Prana is derived from the sun and can be seen as minute, brilliant white specks in the atmosphere. On clear sunny days, there is a vast supply of prana in the atmosphere, which endows us with an abundance of energy, which is why we feel more alive and energetic when the sun shines. On dull, cloudy days the amount of prana is reduced, which can leave us feeling tired and listless. After sunset, prana is greatly decreased, leaving the body to use what it has stored during the day.

Prana embodies seven varieties of energy, each one constituting one of the colours of the spectrum. When prana is absorbed into a human being, it is refracted into the colour spectrum and then each colour is attracted to and absorbed into the relevant major energy centre – or chakra – identified with that colour in the etheric sheath of the aura. From the chakra the colour radiates into the remaining auric layers. (This establishes an important relationship between chakras and the colours – and their vibrational energies – that they channel.)

A major energy centre or chakra is formed where 21 nadis

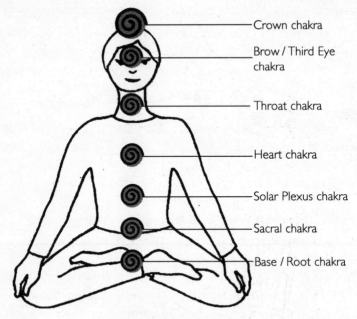

Crown chakra

Brow / Third Eye chakra

Throat chakra

Heart chakra

Solar Plexus chakra

Sacral chakra

Base / Root chakra

Your body and the chakras

cross and there are seven of them, five in line with the physical spine, one situated between the eyebrows and one on top of the head. Each major chakra is connected to one of the endocrine glands in the physical body, thereby playing an important part in therapy, especially if the disease is hormonal in nature. Because both feet and both hands are mirror images of the physical body, the microcosm of the macrocosm, these chakras can also be located along the spinal reflex present on feet and hands. I feel that these points are important for practising reflexologists.

In addition to their associations with the physical body, the chakras, as I have already mentioned, form our spiritual ladder, each one presenting us with the challenges that aid our spiritual growth. As we progress through these challenges, the chakras start to become fully opened, endowing us with their gifts.

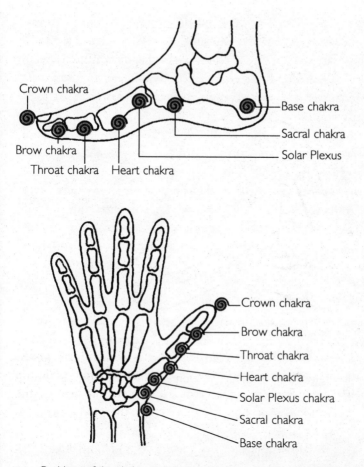

Positions of the chakras on the spinal reflex of the hands and feet

The Base Chakra

The Base chakra, called in Sanskrit the '*Muladhara*', meaning 'root' or 'source', is situated at the perineum. It is related to the element of earth and radiates **red** as its dominant colour. On a physical level, it is identified with the male reproductive organs and with our physical existence.

This chakra holds our instinct for survival, as well as

helping us to keep our feet on the ground. It asks us to look at our physical, earthly existence, how we function as human beings and the care we take of our physical body. This involves learning to listen to our body in order to know what sustenance, rest and exercise it needs. We also need to be firmly rooted to the earth in order to function efficiently on this planet. Our roots are the product of our ancestral conditioning and genetic traits, which can present stumbling blocks for us. The challenge we now face is to look carefully at these roots and to strengthen them by releasing any inherent traits and conditioning that we are still patterning our life on, but which are no longer relevant. Only by doing this are we able to create a strong foundation upon which to build our spiritual life.

The Sacral Chakra

This chakra's Sanskrit name is 'Swadhisthana', meaning 'one's own abode', and it is situated approximately two inches below the navel. It radiates the colour **orange** and is linked to the element of water. On a physical level, it is connected to the female reproductive organs and to the adrenal glands. It also influences the skin, kidneys, bladder, circulatory and lymphatic systems.

All water is symbolic of the Great Mother and associated with the feminine principle. Water is said to be the liquid counterpart of light and the source of all potentialities in existence. Water has the power to dissolve, abolish, purify and regenerate. It is also associated with our emotions, 'the tears of joy or the tears of sorrow'.

Water has the great ability to flow freely when unhindered, therefore the challenge this centre presents is ascertaining whether or not we are flowing with the energies of life. We need to ask ourselves if we are holding on to old emotions that may be hindering us, if we have cleared from our roots the old patterns and genetic traits that act as large boulders, preventing the free flow of all aspects of our being. If we cannot do this, we remain stagnant, failing to allow ourselves to flow with the energies of life. This will ultimately lead to a state of stuckness, which can bring about decay. Sometimes we have to permit ourselves to shed tears of sorrow, anger and pain to dissolve our negative emotions and purify our emotional body to bring about energetic regeneration. Only when we have done this can we climb the ladder to the next chakra.

The Solar Plexus Chakra

Known in Sanskrit as 'Manipura' or 'city of jewels', this chakra is situated just above the navel, approximately between the twelfth thoracic and the first lumbar vertebrae. It radiates **yellow** and is associated with the element of fire and is affiliated to the sun. Here heat is generated, firstly through the process of digestion and secondly through the movement of prana, because this is the centre where prana (the upward-moving vitality) and apana (the downward-moving vitality) meet, creating the heat necessary to sustain life. On a physical level this centre is associated with the stomach, duodenum, gall bladder, liver and pancreas. The endocrine glands with which it is connected are the islets of langerhans, which form part of the pancreas. The Solar Plexus chakra is linked to our emotional life and in highly emotional people is overcharged.

The element that resides here is fire, which purifies and transforms, and on reaching this centre we are ourselves challenged to walk through that fire of purification. This can take many forms and present the many challenges that serve our spiritual growth if we have the courage to face and work with them. The writings of many mystics refer to this time of growth as 'the dark night of the soul', a period when one is unable to see the light through the dark smoke formed from the burning away of our impurities.

Fire is polarised into two complementary aspects of light and heat and the light at this centre is symbolised by the sun. The sun is the heart of the cosmos and symbolic of supreme cosmic power. Dante writes: 'There is no visible thing in all the world more worthy to serve as a symbol of God than the sun that illuminates with visible light, first itself and then all celestial and mundane bodies.' When we emerge from the fire of purification we are reborn into the light of the sun, which nourishes and strengthens us for the continuation of our spiritual journey.

The Heart Chakra

The Heart chakra is situated between the fourth and fifth thoracic vertebrae and radiates the colour **green**. Its Sanskrit name is *'Anahata'*, which translates as 'unstruck'. All universal sound is produced through the striking of objects, which set up vibrations or sound waves. The source of all sound is the primordial sound that comes from beyond this world and manifests at this centre. On a physical level the Heart chakra is connected to the lungs and respiratory system, the heart and circulatory system, the immune system, the arms and hands. The endocrine gland attributed to it is the thymus and the element is air.

This chakra is referred to as the Heart chakra because it is situated slightly to the right of the physical heart and its main attribute is unconditional love. Frequently we talk about our love for fellow human beings, or for the animal and plant kingdoms, but the question we need to ask ourselves is whether this love stems from our intellect or comes unconditionally from our heart. If intellectual, it will bear very little depth and can wither and fade as quickly as it appeared. In order to practise unconditional love, we have to become that love ourselves. This involves loving every part of our physical body, no matter its shape or size, as well as loving our feelings and thoughts. If we are unable to do this, then it is very difficult to love others unconditionally. Unconditional love holds no judgement or criticism, but allows us to accept and love a person regardless of their many faults and idiosyncrasies.

I believe that unconditional love holds the highest vibrational frequency and therefore cannot be contained within itself. It has to flow out to embrace all things that it comes into contact with. At the Heart chakra we are asked to reflect upon our understanding of unconditional love and how we can work towards embracing this in our own life. In the Bible we read that God, the universal creator, is love, the love that is unconditional and embraces all things.

This universal intelligence is also the vital breath of the universe and this is symbolised at this centre by the element of air. Here we are able to breathe in this vital breath, to help with our own spiritual understanding and awareness.

The Throat Chakra

The Sanskrit name of this chakra is '*Vishuddha*', meaning 'to purify'. It is situated between the two clavicle bones and radiates the colour **blue**. Physically this chakra governs the vocal cords, the ears, the nervous system and the female reproductive organs. The endocrine glands linked to it are the thyroid and parathyroids.

The throat centre is complementary to the Sacral chakra in that they are both centres of creativity. The creativity of the Sacral chakra applies mainly to the female principle, because it is involved in the creation of a body for an incarnating soul. The Throat chakra is the centre of higher creativity and resonates with the sounds produced by our vocal cords. The neck represents the bridge between the physical and spiritual life and it is at the Throat chakra that liquid light from the sacral centre is transformed into the brilliant light of the spirit.

To aspire and work with this chakra we have to have our feet firmly on the earth, otherwise we run the risk of becoming so divinely focused that we are no longer physically effective. When we are grounded and have gained mastery over our physical life, this chakra becomes more open. All of this involves patience and the courage to change those things in our life to which we no longer resonate. This can prove difficult because it often creates a sense of insecurity. But once we begin the search for our own inner centre – the place where we find that ultimate peace, security and love that cannot be destroyed – we also find the incentive and courage to continue our journey.

The Brow Chakra

This chakra is located between the two eyebrows at the centre of the brow. Its Sanskrit name is *'Ajna'*, which is translated as 'command'. The colour radiating here is **indigo**. On a physical level it is affiliated to the eyes, nose, ears and brain and the endocrine gland with which it is associated is the pituitary.

The Brow chakra is often depicted as having two petals, symbolising our twofold nature. The challenge we have here is in uniting this twofold nature to wholeness. Our twofold nature is reflected by our ego self and our spirit self; the right and left side of the brain (the intuitive and intellectual) and our masculine and feminine energies. Most esoteric philosophies teach that the Base chakra contains the powerful, latent kundalini energy, referred to as the Shakti, the feminine principle. In the Brow chakra resides the masculine principle, Shiva. When a person is physically, emotionally, mentally and spiritually ready, the Shakti rises through a channel in the etheric sheath, known as the sashumna, which runs parallel to the spine, vivifying all the lower chakras on her way to the Brow chakra. Here she is united with her masculine counterpart Shiva, before rising into the enlightenment of the Crown chakra. This symbology describes how we have to polarise both the negative and positive energies; the masculine and feminine, and the left and right hemispheres of the brain before we can complete our journey into the light of our true spiritual self.

The Crown Chakra

This chakra is found just above the crown of the head. It radiates the colour **violet** and is connected to the pineal gland. Its Sanskrit name is '*Sahasrara*', which is translated as '1,000-petalled lotus', 1,000 being the number of eternity.

This is the centre where our journey ends. Through the many challenges that life has presented and our endeavours to work to overcome them, we finally enter into the state of God Consciousness and become one with that ultimate reality. Our sixth sense has opened, allowing us a feeling of connectedness with both the visible and invisible worlds. We become submerged into that vast ocean of cosmic love, peace and pure bliss. This is the state that we have worked towards through many lifetimes and the place where all the great esoteric paths lead.

The traveller has reached the end of the journey.
In the freedom of the infinite he is free from all sorrows,

the fetters that bound him are thrown away and the
  burning
fever of life is no more.
In the light of his vision he has found his freedom:
his thoughts are peace, his words are peace, his work is
  peace.

The Dhammapada

As well as the seven major chakras, the etheric sheath contains 21 minor chakras formed where 14 nadis cross. The colour that shines from these is a paler shade of the colour emanating from their nearest major chakra. In the head, one is connected to each eye and one to each ear, taking on a shade of indigo. We find one midway along each clavicle and one in the palm of each hand, radiating a pale blue. In the chest a minor chakra is connected to each breast, emanating a shade of green, and one is connected to the thymus, which is turquoise. In the upper abdomen one is connected to the liver and one to the stomach, both taking on a shade of yellow, and two are associated with the spleen, and give off a golden orange. In the lower abdomen there is one near to each gonad, radiating a shade of orange, and in the legs there are ones behind each knee and on the sole of each foot, all radiating red. These chakras are important to work with if a person is suffering a problem in a part of the body that these minor chakras are related to.

EXERCISE: VISUALISATION ON THE CHAKRAS

☆ Sit down in a place that is quiet and warm and where you will not be disturbed. Close your eyes and, starting from your feet and working towards the top of your head, release any tension that you feel present in your physical body.

☆ Relax your mind by looking at the thoughts passing through your mind. Visualise these as beautiful bubbles that gently float into the atmosphere and disperse.

☆ Bring your still and concentrated mind to your spine, making sure that it is straight. Allow your concentration to travel down your spine to its base, the coccyx. It is here that the Base chakra is situated. Imagine this chakra expanding until it is large enough for you to walk inside.

☆ On entering, you find that you are standing in front of a large red tulip. You feel this flower inviting you to come and sit at its centre. You accept this invitation and, sitting quietly, you become aware of the vibrant life energy of the red rays that surround you. In the warm atmosphere that these rays generate, start to contemplate your own life for a while. Are your feet firmly rooted to the earth? Do you need to clear from your life any conditioning or genetic traits that are preventing you from walking forward? If so, how do you propose to do this?

☆ After a few moments of reflection, look to the centre of the tulip and you will find radiating there a beam of white light. Stand up and walk into this light, allowing it to lift you to the Sacral chakra.

☆ At the Sacral chakra you come face to face with a large orange marigold, which also invites you to sit at its centre to become surrounded by the orange rays of light. This colour fills you with energy and joy and gives the sensation of being gently carried on the soft undulating waves of water. Floating and flowing with its movement, are you able to experience the sensations that a dolphin experiences in water: unrestraint, the freedom to swim wherever you wish, exuberant joy and fun, or are you finding rocks and boulders blocking your path? If so, what do these obstacles represent in your life and how can you remove them to procure your freedom? This may be the first time you have become aware of any obstacles or perhaps these have been pushed to the back of your mind because you feel that solving them would be too difficult and painful. Before moving into the next chakra, quietly reflect for a while on what this chakra is saying to you.

☆ When you feel ready, stand up and walk into the white shaft of light emanating from the centre of the marigold, allowing yourself to be gently lifted to the Solar Plexus chakra.

☆ At this centre you stand beside a large yellow sunflower. At its invitation you sit at its centre and become surrounded by yellow rays of light. The sensation that you feel is that of sitting on a sandy beach beneath the brilliance and warmth of the sun's rays. As the warmth of these rays wraps itself around you, contemplate upon 'the fire of purification' and what this means to you personally. Perhaps you have passed through such fires in your life, or maybe this is a stage in your growth that you still have to undergo in order to realise the true splendour of your spiritual sun. Walking through the fire of purification can feel like walking through a long, black, neverending tunnel, but I can assure you that there is light at the tunnel's end, a light that greets with new horizons of hope and love. What is important to remember is that, when passing through this stage, we are never alone. Our guides and the angelic kingdom will always be there to help, if asked.

☆ When you feel ready, stand and walk into the shaft of white light radiating from the centre of this flower, to be lifted into the Heart chakra.

☆ On entering the Heart chakra, you stand before a pale pink rose, the colour of spiritual, unconditional love. You are invited to sit at its centre and surround yourself with the protective orb of spiritual love that this colour gives. Sitting and relaxing, start to think about unconditional love. Consider whether or not you are able to love all aspects of yourself, as well as all those whom you contact, without judgement or criticism. This means loving their imperfections alongside their irritating habits. Until we are able to fully and unconditionally love ourselves, it is very difficult to unconditionally love others. Love has a broad spectrum, ranging from lust at one end to unconditional love at the other. Where along this spectrum do you feel that you stand?

☆ When you have allowed yourself time to contemplate the spiritual lesson that this centre holds, find the shaft of white light to continue your journey to the Throat chakra.

☆ At the Throat chakra, you find a large blue cornflower that is bidding you sit at its centre, where it will surround you with a blue cloak of peace, relaxation and protection. Remember that this centre represents the bridge that we have to cross in order to pass from the physical into the spiritual realm. Do you feel ready to cross this bridge? If not, you can remain here, wrapped in your blue cloak of protection and peace.

☆ If you feel ready to continue your journey, first contemplate the following lines from the Chandogya Upanishad:

> To one who goes over this bridge, the night
>   becomes like unto day;
> because in the worlds of the spirit, there is a light
>   which is everlasting.

Have you ever thought about the spirit world? If so, do you believe in it? The spiritual journey that we have embarked upon must ultimately give us insight into this world and also to that everlasting light. You may feel that the time is now right for you to explore this realm further and if this is so, there are many excellent books on this subject on the market.

☆ If you are continuing your journey, stand and walk into the shaft of light coming from the centre of the cornflower to be lifted to the Brow chakra. If you feel that you are not ready to continue, stay surrounded by the peace and protection of your blue cloak until you feel ready to end this visualisation.

☆ At the Brow chakra lives a deep indigo iris. When you enter and sit at the iris's centre, the indigo light creates for you the vision of infinite space, which initially seems to be filled with total silence, but as you listen the most wonderful harmonious, undulating sounds reach your ears. These are the sounds made by each planet and star that lives in the universe. These heavenly bodies are never silent. Each one is continuously harmonising with the sound of its neighbour.

☆ If you listen very carefully, you will hear another sound, the voice of your own intuition. Listen to what it is telling you, and ask any questions that you are seeking the answers to. Don't be disappointed if you do not receive an answer immediately, but remember – when you are ready to know, the answer will come. When we first encounter the vastness of space represented in this colour, it can create a certain amount of fear or apprehension, but when we have discovered and become one with our own divinity this fear is replaced by great joy and peace because we have gained the realisation that this vast cosmic space is part of us and we are part of it.

☆ With these thoughts in mind, enter the shaft of light that rises from the centre of the iris, so that you may be lifted to the Crown chakra.

☆ As you enter this chakra, you stand before a many-faceted diamond. Each face of the diamond represents one aspect of yourself. Note that some of the faces are bright and shiny; others are dusty and dull. Also reflected in this precious stone is your own spirituality, the progress that you have made along your chosen path. Sitting quietly, look into the diamond, and listen to what it has to say to you.

☆ When you feel ready, begin your journey back to earth consciousness passing back through each of the chakras and your awareness of their colours. Start by increasing your inhalation and exhalation. Imagine the flower at each chakra closing back to a bud, until you finally visualise a clear red light radiating from your Base chakra, down your legs and feet, anchoring you back to the earth plane. Lastly, open your eyes.

☆ This meditation can be practised as a whole or each of the chakras can be individually meditated upon.

The Emotional (or Astral) Body

The emotional or astral body forms the third sheath of the aura, interpenetrating with both the physical and the etheric. The colours displayed here are a reflection of our feelings. Negative emotions such as anger or fear create imbalances resulting in this part of the aura vibrating to the wrong frequency. Because all the layers of the aura interpenetrate, a wrong frequency in this layer will adversely affect all the other layers. If not rectified it will eventually manifest as a physical disease. This principle applies to each of the auric sheaths. If you become emotionally upset, visualise a bright clear yellow coming from the earth, into your feet and legs and into the Solar Plexus chakra. Continue to do this until you feel calm and relaxed.

The Lower Mental Body

This forms the fourth layer of the aura and is connected to our thought patterns. Every thought that we have creates a form or shape. These accumulate in the mental body and can be projected into the environment, surrounding us with thought forms that we and other individuals have created. If a person is sensitive, they are able to detect these thought forms; this is one explanation why a person may suddenly think about a friend minutes before they telephone. Absent healing works on this principle. If someone asks us to send healing, the process of thinking of the person and the colours that would be most beneficial for them creates and projects those colours through the formation of our created thought forms.

It is said that like attracts like, and this is very true. If a person holds very negative attitudes, these will attract thought forms of a similar nature, thereby amplifying their negativity. The same applies for someone who has a very positive outlook on life. This knowledge should help us to be aware of our thoughts, endeavouring to change negative ones into positive.

The Higher Mental Body

This comprises the fifth layer of the aura and is the voice of our intuition or higher self. Through this layer we are taught by our higher self and guided through our difficulties. The voice of the intuition is always correct, although at times the information received can seem unrealistic. If a person chooses to become a channel for healing, especially colour healing, they have to learn to listen to and trust the information they receive from this source. When working with colour therapy, there are specific colours for certain diseases, but each individual is unique so some people may need a different colour than the one prescribed. If we are in tune with our intuition, we will instinctively know the correct colour to give. This is just one example of the necessity of learning to work with our intuition.

The Causal Body

This embodies the sixth layer of the aura and contains the cause for our present earthly incarnation, plus a record of all previous lives. When we incarnate, we choose the parents and the place that will provide the best environment for our spiritual growth and for paying off our chosen karma. Karma is the law of cause and effect that teaches that whatever good you do will be repaid with good and that whatever evil you do will lead to retribution. Jesus Christ explained karma by saying that whatever you sow, so you will reap. When we incarnate, it is the soul's intention to remember the tasks that it has come to fulfil. Unfortunately, because of conditioning, we forget these tasks. It is rather like setting out on a journey and leaving the map behind. Sometimes, in moments of silence, we are able to access the causal body and gain insight and inspiration on the way forward. The colours seen in this layer are ethereal and depend upon our ability to follow the path we have chosen in life.

The Bodyless Body

This forms the seventh layer of the aura and is our 'true essence', that divine spark without beginning or ending. Very few people's auric sight is sufficiently open to 'see' this part of the aura, but it is reputed to be filled with white light. The brilliance and extent of this light depends upon our spiritual growth. In yoga, one of the questions a student is asked to ask themselves is 'Who am I?' The answer they frequently give is their first name, the name given to the physical body. But, if their first name is taken away, what then is the answer to the question?

The search for our divine self can take many lifetimes and

starts with the discipline of meditation and study of one of the esoteric paths. One encouraging thought: whatever point in our search for self we have reached at the end of any lifetime, we always start our next life from that point.

EXERCISE: FILLING THE AURA WITH COLOUR

☆ Sit down in a place that is quiet and warm, where you will not be disturbed. Close your eyes and, starting from your feet and working towards the top of your head, release any tension that you feel present in your physical body. Check to make sure that your spine is straight.

☆ Relax your mind by looking at the thoughts that are passing through, visualising these as beautiful bubbles that gently float into the atmosphere and disperse.

☆ Bring your concentration to the crown of your head where you will see a ray of white light from the cosmos entering. This ray of light is always present. It is our connection to the spiritual realm. Visualise this ray of light travelling from your head, down through your body to your feet. Upon reaching your feet it enters into the sacred darkness of the earth, where it becomes refracted into the seven colours of the spectrum. Imagine these colours streaming back through your feet and into your body. As this rainbow of light flows through the major chakras, see each one becoming vivified with its own vibrational colour. When the light spectrum reaches your head it becomes transformed back to white light.

☆ Continue to practise this exercise for approximately 10 minutes. Allow your body to become re-energised with the wonderful colours that form part of our being.

4

The Vibrational Energies of Colour

Colour is a vital force. It is a manifestation of the Divine Mind. It is the original cosmic vibration.

Anonymous

Colour is a living energy whose power affects us physically, emotionally, mentally and spiritually. The colours radiating through our aura are made manifest by our thoughts, feelings, physical health and spiritual development. People gifted with auric sight are able to see energy blocks present in the auric field and, depending upon their degree of development, can assess whether these energy stagnations arise from the emotional, mental or spiritual sheath and how these blocked energies will eventually affect the physical body, if not dissolved.

Colour is perceived either as light (illuminatory colour) or pigment (solid colour derived from dyes). Of these two forms, light has the most profound effect upon cellular structure and for this reason is used in therapy, though illuminatory colour can have contra-indications and therefore should only be used by qualified colour practitioners. When using colour for self-help, the use of pigment colour is always recommended.

The Spectrum

Each colour has its own spectrum, ranging from the palest to the darkest shade. The paler shades are produced by adding white and the darker shades by adding black to the spectral colour. Colours carry both negative and positive attributes. Bright, clear shades denote the positive qualities and dull, muddy shades the negative. For example, a vibrant green in the aura shows a balanced and relaxed state, but a dark, gloomy green indicates avarice and envy.

A person's like or dislike of a particular colour can depend on its use – whether, for example, it is used for decoration, in art, or in clothing. When worn, one major consideration is the colour's ability to enhance skin tone and hair colouring. Another is the overall feeling that the colour inspires. In decoration, more than one colour is used, so the general effect that the colours produce becomes the main criteria. Dislike of a colour also has a wide range of causes. This again can be purely cosmetic – the colour does not suit us, or we do not look good dressed in it – though it can also stem from a deep psychological root, as when a child is subjected to unpleasant or frightening experiences. What often makes an impression on the child is the colour of the clothes worn by the perpetrator, which then becomes associated with pain or fear. As the child matures, the experiences becomes locked away in the unconscious mind, but the conscious mind retains the dislike of the colour without knowing the reason. To uncover the cause, counselling or regression therapy is used to bring the experience back to the conscious mind, where it can be examined and worked with. This ultimately leads to acceptance of the colour.

The fashion industry also has a great influence on the colours that we wear. When the new season's colours appear on the market, we are conditioned to buy clothes in these shades so as not to appear outdated and lacking in fashion sense. Unfortunately, these so-called fashionable colours are seldom the ones that we need therapeutically. I personally have experienced great difficulty in buying clothes in the colours that I want if they are out of fashion. When we begin to explore and understand the vibrational frequencies of colour and the part that these energies play in our well-being, our sensitivity to colour heightens. This endows us with the knowledge of the colour we therapeutically need at any given time. With this heightened sensitivity, there is a tendency to keep in one's wardrobe at least one garment in each of the spectral colours. I am very happy to say, at this stage in our development, we are no longer so conditioned or dictated to by the fashion industry.

I envisage colour as a many-faceted diamond. The central facet radiates white light, which bathes its surrounding facets in the many hues of colour contained within itself. I also see the rainbow not in two-dimensional form as portrayed in books but in three-dimensional form, creating a tube of colour from the centre of which white light radiates. Where the red and violet light meet on this tube, the beautiful colour of magenta appears.

In colour therapy, a practitioner may choose to work with eight or ten colours or with the twelve colours that form the tertiary colour wheel. But, regardless of the number of colours used, a complementary colour must always be used alongside the treatment colour, because the one has been found to balance the other. To find the complementary colour, look at the diagram of the ten-colour wheel. Select one of its colours and then look diagonally opposite across the wheel to find its complementary colour. For example, the complementary colour of blue is orange. When working with pigment colour, it is not so imperative to use the complementary colour.

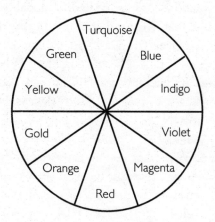

The ten-colour wheel

The information and exercises given in this book will be based on the seven spectral colours of red, orange, yellow, green, blue, indigo and violet, with the addition of magenta. It is important to first learn about and work with the basic colour spectrum before extending to the tertiary colours.

The diagram on page 54 pictures a many-faceted diamond. The central facet is radiating white light. The 32 facets surrounding the central facet are divided into eight sections of four facets. Each of the eight sections relate to one of the spectral colours of red, orange, yellow, green, blue, indigo, violet or magenta, and each of the four facets contained within each section vibrates to a different shade of its prescribed colour. The darkest shade represents the physical body and the lightest shade the spiritual. The two shades in between stand for the emotional body (the darker shade) and the mental body (the lighter shade). You might enjoy colouring this in the appropriate colours.

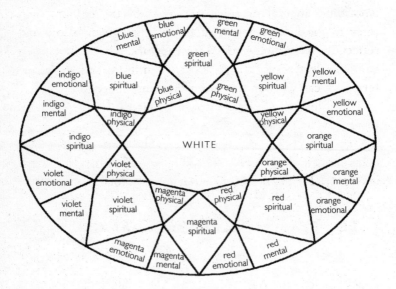

A many-faceted diamond

To work with these colours you will need to obtain 32 short lengths of ribbon (approximately 8 inches long) comprising the eight colours. Each of the eight main colours contains four ribbons of different shades. The darkest shade of each ribbon will represent the physical body, the lightest shade the spiritual and the two in-between shades the emotional and mental. To make things easier, you might like to mark each of the four shades: P for physical, E for emotional, M for mental and S for spiritual. When you have collected your ribbons you can either make a simple white bag in cotton or linen to put them in or you can keep them in a carrier bag. When they are in the bag, mix them up and then, without looking, place your hand into the bag and ask your higher self to select a ribbon you currently need. When you have singled out your ribbon, look to see if you have chosen the physical, emotional, mental or spiritual aspect of the colour, then refer to the interpretation of the colours given below and reflect on its meaning for you. To work with your chosen colour, select one of the methods given in the ensuing chapters. You can work in this way with your ribbons daily.

The colour that we select or a colour that we feel drawn towards is an indication that we are lacking one or more of the qualities afforded to that colour. The chosen colour also helps us to look at ourselves to discover the changes that we need to make in our lives in order to walk forward.

The Properties of the Eight Colours

Red

On the electromagnetic spectrum, red is at the heat end of the spectrum, falling next to infra-red. This colour relates to the vibrant, sometimes aggressive masculine energy. It is the symbol of life, strength and vitality, therefore a very powerful energiser and stimulant. Red has the ability to increase the flow of blood in the physical body and, for this reason, people suffering high blood pressure, hypertension or heart disease should not be subjected to red light. It is also a colour that helps us to stay grounded, especially if we are in danger of becoming so heavenly minded we are no earthly good. We incarnated into the earth for a reason; to fulfil this purpose it is essential that we create a balance in our physical and spiritual life.

The negative energies associated with red are lust, anger and aggression.

Physical: Choosing red on a physical level could be for a number of reasons. Firstly it could indicate that you lack physical energy, perhaps because of a hard day's work. But, because all aspects of our being are inter-related, the tiredness could also stem from emotional or mental trauma, the cause of which needs to be recognised and worked with in order to cure the symptom. Perhaps your choice of this colour is a sign that you need to ground your energies. It is a common occurrence for people starting along a spiritual path to neglect their earthly connection. Remember, it is important to stay grounded for the integration of the spiritual and earthly energies. If by nature you are a person who feels the cold, you may be drawn to red for its warmth. In Victorian times, when heating was restricted to one room, it was customary to wear a red flannel night shirt, believing that this would help to sustain the body's heat. Your selection of red may also indicate that you suffer low blood pressure. Red is the main colour given therapeutically for this condition.

Emotional: Here the choice of red indicates a lack of emotional energy, which nearly always suggests the presence of emotional problems or trauma. These problems may not necessarily refer specifically to you but to a loved one. Working with red will give you the energy to face and find the solution to your own problems and the courage to help loved ones and friends through their difficulties.

Mental: If you need this colour mentally, it is showing that you are mentally tired. If caused by intellectual hard work, this is remedied by a good night's sleep. If this is not the cause, then red is inviting you to look at your personal life, because mental tiredness can be linked to personal problems that constantly churn over in our minds in search of an answer. Working with red on a regular basis will give you the energy to find and work with the solution resulting in you being able to see your way forward.

Spiritual: When we start to work with our spirituality through, for example, meditation or a religious discipline, it is very easy to segregate this newly found path from the routine of daily life. If you have found this happening to you, then working with red will help you to integrate your spiritual and physical life. It is very easy to initially become so absorbed in heavenly pursuits that we become physically useless. If this happens, the spiritual realm has ways of putting hurdles on our path to bring us down to earth.

Orange

This is also an energising colour but, unlike red, it contains the gentle, caring properties of the feminine energy. Although not complementary in colour to red, it is complementary to its energies, red being aligned with the masculine energy and orange with the feminine. Orange is a colour that enhances our creative talents and generates joy because of its ability to change biochemical structure, resulting in the dispersal of depression. Its negative attributes are pride and a leaning towards being over-ambitious.

Physical: Feeling drawn to orange physically could be symptomatic of a lack of energy, depression or a female disorder. If you feel that it is associated with low energy or depression, then working with orange will help the symptoms while you find and work with the cause. If it is connected to a female disorder, then it is advisable to seek a medical diagnosis and work with orange alongside medical advice. Another reason for the need for this colour could be the lack of use of your own creativity and intuition. Our brain has left and right hemispheres and, if we are to function as a whole being, we need to work with both. The left hemisphere is connected to our intellect and the right to our intuition and creativity. If our career is intellectually demanding, we need to choose a creative hobby, and vice versa.

Emotional: If you have singled out orange emotionally it is indicating a lack of emotional joy in your life. The cause could be twofold. It could be identified with an emotional problem that is not being resolved, present or in the past. Or it may be associated with a relationship, or lack of one. A relationship has to feel right if we are to receive and give the affection and nurturing so essential for our well-being. While working with this colour, take time to reflect on these aspects of your life to discover if there are any that need working with.

Mental: Being attracted mentally to this colour implies a lack of mental joy. The cause could be an uninspiring job or, in a woman, it could result from giving up a fulfilling and exciting career in order to raise a family. A lack of mental joy is associated with depression, of which the causes are many: the weather, an uninteresting task that needs to be tackled or the all-work-and-no-play syndrome. If you are suffering any of the above, work with orange, but also aim to find ways of bringing mental stimulation and joy into your life.

Spiritual: If you have selected orange on a spiritual level, it is challenging you to look at your own beliefs. Are you following a religious dogma that no longer holds any truth for you, but conditioning prevents you from letting go and moving forward? If the answer is yes, the challenge you are facing is to find the courage to follow what you believe, stepping aside from all things that do not pertain to that. I personally believe that all religions and disciplines contain part of the ultimate truth and, as we spiritually mature, it may be necessary to change direction many times.

Yellow

Yellow is the colour nearest to natural daylight and its rays carry positive magnetic colours that are inspiring and stimulating. Frequently people who spend much of their life indoors are attracted towards this colour. Although yellow has many beneficial qualities, it can never replace natural daylight and the message it conveys to the people it attracts is that more time needs to be spent outdoors. This colour strengthens the nervous system and stimulates the motor nerves in the physical body, which then produce energy in the muscles. It helps calcium metabolism and skin problems, making the vibrational energy of yellow beneficial for healing arthritis, skin disorders, broken bones and scar tissue. The malign aspect of yellow is its connotation with cowardice.

Physical: If you have selected the yellow ribbon relating to your physical body, check the physical disorders given above for this colour to see if they are relevant to you. If not, could it relate to you needing to spend more time outdoors? The ultra-violet rays found in natural daylight are essential for our well-being and this essential ingredient is often lacking in modern life-styles. Endeavour to spend at least 30 minutes outdoors each day, removing contact lenses or spectacles.

Yellow also holds the property of detachment and on this level questions our adeptness to separate ourselves from our physical bodies. A typical case of this would be someone continually looking in the mirror to make sure that their clothes, hair and make-up are in impeccable order. The lesson that needs to be learned from this is that beauty comes from within and not from without. If we meet a person who is badly deformed but functioning from their spiritual self, the beauty that shines through their eyes detracts from their physical deformity. While working with the light of this colour, try looking at yourself with the thoughts given above in mind.

Emotional: This colour frequently reveals itself on an emotional level to help us to step aside from our feelings in order to view them in a new light and to handle them more efficiently. It also assists us to stand back when working therapeutically with others. This is vital in its prevention of emotional involvement with them or their problems. To become emotionally attached to clients would help neither them nor us. If you are currently faced with an emotional issue that has more than one solution, write down the pros and cons of each. This allows you to see which solution has the most positive attributes and therefore helps to provide the answer. You might try using yellow paper for this exercise!

Mental: If this colour has come up for you mentally, it could be an indication that you are mentally overtaxed and need to relax for a while. You also need to ask yourself if the cause of your mental tiredness results from the constant churning of unsolved problems in your mind, which does not always supply the answer. The act of standing back and surveying your thoughts often throws light on the situation, resulting in the right solution being found. Working with yellow through visualisation prior to doing this can be of great help. Yellow, the colour connected to the intellect, frequently appears in the aura around the heads of people lecturing or engaged in intellectual pusuits. As it is connected with the intellect, it is a very good colour to have in a study.

Spiritual: In spiritual matters, this colour can be aligned with a doubting Thomas, someone who reads or hears spiritual truths but is always trying to prove them intellectually. This makes it very difficult for an intellectual to learn to listen to and trust their intuition. Our intuition always speaks truth, but the knowledge it imparts cannot always be proven. When this colour appears spiritually, it can speak to a person of trust to follow what they intuitively feel is right. Having selected this colour spiritually, do its attributes ring true for you? If so, perhaps the time is now right for you to start trusting and being guided by your intuition. Working with meditation on a regular basis is invaluable in this quest.

Green

Green is the colour of balance, and works with our duality. It lies at the centre of the spectrum and is the colour that is focused directly on to the retina by the lens of the eyes, bringing them relaxation, which is then transmitted to the rest of the body. This is why the greens of nature are able to induce in us a state of relaxation. Another form of its duality is its association with both life and decay. As life, it appears with the new foliage of spring; as its negative aspect, decay, it is the colour of the mould found on rotting vegetation.

As human beings, we comprise body, mind and spirit, and contain both feminine and masculine, positive and negative energies. In order to become whole, this duality in our nature has to be united, and this can take many lifetimes to achieve.

The negative qualities associated with green are envy, jealousy and nausea.

Physical: Choosing green on a physical level may be indicative of an imbalance in the physical body, often caused by disease or surgical intervention. When this imbalance occurs, the rest of the body will compensate to keep the whole in homeostasis. This colour could also be trying to tell you that the emotional or mental layer of your aura is vibrating to the wrong frequency, creating an overall imbalance, in which case the cause needs to be found and worked with. While you work with the cause, visualising green entering the Throat Chakra will help to cleanse and maintain the aura's correct frequency. Green, the dominant colour of the Heart chakra, makes it a strong colour for balancing the energies of the heart and lungs.

Emotional: If you are drawn to this colour on an emotional level, it usually indicates emotional suffering, leading to an imbalance in the astral layer of the aura. The cause for this is usually related to fear, anger, jealousy or hatred that needs to be worked with. The emotional layer of the aura can become blocked, with the stagnated energy arising from old emotional patterns that are no longer relevant but have not been cleared. Hanging on to these dead emotions prevents us from walking forward and evolving spiritually. It is similar to cramming the attic so full of junk that the light from the window is blocked out. This lack of light prevents us from seeing our way clearly. Quietly reflect on these thoughts, examining their relevance to you.

Mental: Selecting green on a mental level shows a lack of mental balance. This could refer to mental instability, but it is more likely to indicate an imbalance in the left and right hemispheres of the brain brought about by working purely with the intellect or solely with creative pursuits. To restore the balance between these two hemispheres requires work with both our intellect and creativity equally. If you are intellectually inclined, take up a creative hobby; if creatively biased, find an interesting way to work with your intellect.

Spiritual: Opting for green spiritually implies spiritual imbalance and requires us to look at our beliefs. This requires us to question any dogma or conditioning that we still veer towards, examining its continuing validity and the possibility of letting go of it. This exercise could be called a spiritual spring-clean. Allowing outdated dogma and conditioning to rule our lives is similar to putting on blinkers, which allow us to see only part of the truth, never the whole truth. When we have become one with that ultimate reality or God, dogma fails to exist, because we are now able to see truth in all things.

Blue

Blue is a colour that veers towards the cold end of the spectrum, symbolising inspiration, peace and tranquillity. It has the ability to expand space and slow down vibrational frequencies, which makes it a good colour to use in a healing or meditation room. It is also an excellent colour if you are suffering tension, high blood pressure, insomnia and stress. Its negative aspect lies in its ability to cause depression and sadness, making it unsuitable for use on anyone suffering these complaints. This colour's calming attributes make it a wonderful colour to wear during pregnancy. It is important to realise that any colour worn during this time will affect the foetus.

Physical: Needing blue physically could imply that you are suffering stress, tension or physical tiredness. Physical tiredness could be due to a day's hard work and will be remedied with a good night's sleep. Stress and tension could also be related to an emotional problem, in which case the cause needs to be identified and found. High blood pressure, or/and insomnia, may be other reasons for your choice, and mean you should work with the colour blue on a regular basis.

Emotional: Picking blue on the emotional level points to stress and tension in this area of your life. Emotional stress is triggered by fear, anger, depression and aggression. If this rings true for you, working with blue will create an emotional state of peace and stillness that will enable you to look at these feelings. If the stress is caused through caring for a loved one who is sick, blue will give you the strength and peace to continue. What I have found interesting in working with students is that they fail to acknowledge emotional stress until it is brought to their attention through their attraction to this colour. This has taught me that colour, as well as being a great healer, is also a great teacher.

Mental: Selecting blue mentally indicates a need for mental peace and relaxation. Mental stress can be brought about by overworking the intellect, which can happen when we have a very demanding career or when we are studying. It can also arise when we are trying to solve problems related to everyday living. Mental overstimulation can lead to insomnia. If you suffer this, work with blue before retiring for the night.

Spiritual: Spiritually blue is the colour of peace and devotion. It is the dominant colour of the Throat chakra, which forms the bridge between the physical and spiritual realms. An attraction to blue spiritually asks us to define our understanding of spirituality. It makes us question whether we are following the spiritual path that is right for us now and also makes us look at where we stand on that bridge and to seek the way that helps us forward in our spiritual life.

Indigo

Indigo is created with blue and violet, making it an inspirational colour. Its blue content speaks of peace and the violet of the spiritual aspirations that lead to unconditional love. This colour is purported to have the ability to psychologically clear and clean the psychic currents of the body. It is also a powerful painkiller and is claimed to have a powerful effect on mental complaints. Its negative attributes revolve around its ability to encourage isolation, depression and solitude.

Physical: If you are drawn towards indigo physically, it is an indication that you need to create recreational space for yourself. Ideally this should occur on a daily basis, but the pressures of modern life do not always allow for this. If impossible on a daily basis, try to set aside an afternoon or a day each week to do whatever you enjoy. Another reason for picking this colour is for physical pain. If you have suffered this for some time, you should seek a medical diagnosis. Never try to eliminate pain with colour without knowing the cause.

Emotional: On an emotional level, the need for indigo usually indicates emotional stress and tension. Here space is requested for the careful examination and assessment of the state of the emotional self and finding ways to solve existing problems.

Mental: Needing indigo mentally is the colour's way of showing that you need mental space. Our brain can get tired from excessive use in the same way as our physical body. Mental space can be created through sleep or meditation. With practice, the whole of life can become a meditation, creating a continuous state of serenity and peace for the mind.

Spiritual: At a spiritual level, indigo is expressing the need for you to find your own inner space, where dwells ultimate peace, truth and security. Finding this place allows us to stand complete within ourselves and feel at home in any place or situation. Working with indigo in meditation and visualisation will help in this quest but it will take time, especially if these ideas are new to you.

Violet

Violet contains the vibrant red masculine energy and the peaceful calm feminine energy of blue. Because this colour contains both these energies, it has the power to balance them within a human person. Violet teaches us self-respect, dignity and self-love. It has been found by those researching the field of colour that emotionally immature and insecure people tend to be attracted towards violet.

Its negative attributes relate to power, manipulation and sexual abuse.

Physical: If you are needing violet physically, ask yourself if you are able to love your physical body, regardless of its shape, size or condition. If the answer is no, then you have to search for the reason why. The underlying cause could be the result of conditioning or that you feel your body is unattractive. An exercise that helps is to look into a mirror before going to bed and on rising each morning and saying to your reflection, 'I love you, I love you, I love you.' You may laugh at this suggestion, but I can assure you that it works. Unfortunately, certain religious teachings suggest that the body is sinful and should be despised. St Francis of Assisi always referred to his body as Brother Ass. This I find very sad, because the physical body is the temple for the soul, whose radiance and beauty is reflected through the eyes.

Emotional: If you have chosen the ribbon relating to the emotional aspect of this colour it challenges you to look at your feelings to discover if you are able to love and respect them, regardless of whether they take on a negative or positive form. Working with violet allows us to look at our anger or jealousy, find its source and respectfully attempt to eradicate it. Development in this way helps us to grow in love and respect for ourselves.

Mental: Needing this colour mentally invites us to assess our ability to love what we are thinking, accepting our thoughts as part of our self. This is especially difficult if we are prone to negativity, but as we grow to love and accept ourselves as human and spiritual beings, so our thoughts and feelings will change to become more positive and harmonious. In all of this work, one of the things that I have found essential is a good sense of humour. A capacity to laugh at ourselves is half the battle.

Spiritual: If you are spiritually attracted to violet, it is challenging you to contemplate the concept of unconditional love. Unconditional love is a state where we are able to love all things, regardless of their physical, mental or emotional state. To be able to do this, I believe that we ourselves first have to become unconditional love; when we have reached this state, we no longer have to think whether or not we love a person, we do it automatically. Unconditional love is free from judgement, so the first step is to be aware of our judgement of others and the second step is learning to transform this into love.

Magenta

Magenta comprises the colours red and violet. On the electro-magnetic spectrum, red lies next to infra-red and violet next to ultra-violet, giving this ray a burning, cutting quality. Magenta is therefore a colour that we can work with to cut through or cut out of our lives those things that are no longer relevant, such as a past relationship to which we are still emotionally tied, or foods that we are addicted to but that hold no nutritional value. It is only by eradicating such things from our lives that change can take place. It is similar to removing a river dam to allow the water to flow freely. The process of letting go and changing can be painful and uncom-fortable, but all journeys that are worth taking bear some discomfort. The joy comes when we see a clear road ahead. The negative qualities of this colour are manipulation and a sense of self-worthlessness, sometimes coupled with inner anger.

Physical: If you are attracted to this colour on a physical level, it could mean that you need to change a physical activi-ty. This could be connected to a career, home or leisure pastime, or even the colour of the clothes that you wear. You may love to wear black, believing this to be a chic, fashionable and slimming colour; maybe so, but black attracts all things to itself, including negativity from other people, and this may now be the time to bring more colour into your wardrobe and into your life. As you increase your colour sensitivity, you should find yourself drawn towards colours that you need therapeutically. These are the colours that you need to work with.

Emotional: When we are drawn to magenta emotionally, it is asking us to step aside from our feelings to find and eradicate those belonging to the past. If we hope to progress in life, we have to let go of the past. It has gone and we cannot change it. We can review it, carry forward its positive aspects, learn from its mistakes – and then let go. This is a difficult task for many people, because they look upon their failings as a sin. I regard mistakes as lessons. If we learn from them then the past is healed.

Mental: If you have chosen magenta on a mental level, it is asking you to look at and release old thought patterns. A case could be a person who is constantly referring back to the good old days. I believe that all days are good if looked at in the right spirit. When you start to look consciously at what you are thinking, I am sure that you will be surprised at the amount of negativity present. Working with magenta allows these negative thoughts to be gently changed to positive ones.

Spiritual: Spiritually, magenta is showing us that it is time to move forward in our spiritual life. The earth colour of red and the spiritual colour of violet have united to form the next evolutionary spiral. If we ask for guidance from the spiritual realm and the angelic kingdoms, we will be shown what we

69

need to do to take the next step on this spiral of life. A great aid on our spiritual journey is visualisation. If we are able to visualise every day, the next step that we intuitively feel is right, the way becomes smoother and progress is faster.

Working with these colours on a regular basis gives great insight into ourself and teaches us many things.

5

Working with the Chakras and Their Colours Through Yoga

Yoga is a darsana
a mirror to look at ourselves from within.
Control of the mind is yoga,
when the mind is stilled and silenced,
what remains is the soul.
It is the request of the soul, the spark of divinity within us
which is the very purpose of yoga.

B.K.S. Iyengar

Colour is worked with in yoga through the postures and their relevant chakras, each of the classical postures dealing with one or more of the seven main chakras. Chapter 3 describes how these chakras each radiate one of the colours of the spectrum and influence the endocrine glands and bodily functions attributed to it.

By focusing on the relevant chakra and visualising the living energy of the colour flooding the chakra and radiating into the aura when holding a posture, the benefits afforded to the posture will be greatly increased, any energy stagnation in the chakra will be cleared and, if it is a posture working with your chosen colour, you will also be working with your need for that colour. You can also work systematically with each of the postures and their accompanying colours. Doing this will help keep your body healthy and strong and increase your colour awareness and sensitivity. To derive maximum benefit from a posture it has to be held for as long as possible in preference to repeating the posture several times.

The Practice of Yoga

Little is known about the origin of yoga except that it is believed to have come from the Indus Valley. Archaeological excavations at Mahenjo Daro in the Indus Valley in 1922, uncovered faience seals, dated to the third millennium BC, which depicted men sitting in full lotus posture with their eyes closed in meditation. On either side of these meditators stood a worshipper with folded hands and behind each worshipper was a half-reared snake. In yogic philosophy, the snake symbolises the latent energy that resides in the Base chakra. When the aspirant is ready emotionally, mentally and physically, the serpent rises through the susumna, the main channel situated inside the spinal column, piercing the seven main chakras on its path to the Crown chakra. At this chakra it is released through the top of the head, bringing about samadhi, or enlightenment.

The word yoga is derived from the Sanskrit word 'yuj', meaning to yoke, join or unite. Its aim is the achievement of God-consciousness through the integration of all aspects of our being. This makes yoga a discipline, a way of life. Yoga is one of the six orthodox systems of Indian philosophy. It was systematised by an Eastern seer Patanjali in his classical work, the *Yoga Sutras*, laying down the eight steps or limbs of yoga that have to be followed in order to obtain enlightenment. These are:

1. The Yamas (universal moral commandments)
2. The Niyamas (self-purification by discipline)
3. Asana (posture)
4. Pranayama (rhythmic control of the breath)
5. Pratyahara (sense withdrawal)
6. Dharna (concentration)
7. Dhyana (meditation)
8. Samadhi (God-consciousness)

One of the most important authorities on yoga philosophy is the Bhagavad Gita, where Sri Krishna explains to Arjuna the meaning of yoga as a deliverance from contact with pain and sorrow:

> When the mind of the yogi is in harmony and finds rest in the spirit within, all restless desires gone, then he is a Yukta, one in God. Then his soul is a lamp whose light is steady, for it burns in a shelter where no winds come. When the mind is resting in the stillness of the prayer of yoga, and by the grace of the spirit sees the spirit and therein finds fulfilment; then the seeker knows the joy of eternity: a vision seen by reason far beyond what senses can see. He abides therein and moves not from truth. He has found the treasure above all others. There is nothing higher than this. He who has achieved it shall not be moved by the greatest sorrow. This is the real meaning of yoga – a deliverance from contact with pain and sorrow.

In the West, the third limb of yoga, asana, is the one most widely known, though it is most frequently taught as a keep-fit routine. In fact the real importance of the asanas lies in their ability to increase the flow of energy in the physical body and to strengthen it in preparation for the powerful flow of energy generated from yogic practices. This can only be achieved if the position of the posture and the breathing that accompanies it is correct. When practising the classical asanas of yoga, each one should embrace within itself all of the eight steps set out by Patanjali. For example, if one strains the physical body when practising the postures then the first yama, which is non-violence, is not being adhered to; the correct breathing should accompany the posture, and the whole concentration should be centred on the posture throughout its duration, not allowing extraneous noises to distract one's concentration. Having achieved this, the asana becomes a meditation able to lift one on to a higher level of consciousness.

In order to reap the benefits offered by yoga, practice must be regular. This also applies when working with yoga in conjunction with colour. When practising yoga, it is advisable to set aside the same time each day. This creates a good habit and makes your practice something to look forward to, especially when you start to experience renewed energy and a greater sense of well-being. Yoga should be practised on an empty stomach. If you practise the first yama on a full stomach, you could upset the digestive system, which would, in yoga terms, be a violation against the physical body. Wear loose clothing to allow free and easy movement, and always start your session with a short relaxation to centre yourself and quieten the mind. If your body is stiff, extend only into the posture to the point where discomfort is felt. With practice, the muscles will become supple, allowing you to complete the full posture. At the end of your practice session, lie down, cover yourself with a blanket and relax. During this relaxation time, feel into your body for any changes that may have occurred. Visualise each of your chakras vibrating with colour and your aura clothing you in a coat of many vibrant colours. While you are relaxing, you might like to contemplate these words spoken by Sri Krishna to Arjuna:

> Yoga is a harmony. Not for him who eats too much, or for him who eats too little; nor for him who sleeps too little, or for him who sleeps too much. A harmony in eating and resting, in sleeping and keeping awake: a perfection in whatever one does. This is the yoga that gives peace from all pain.

If you reap benefit from practising the yoga asanas given in this book, you may wish to learn more about the subject, in which case I suggest that you attend a yoga class run by a qualified teacher. It is very difficult to learn yoga from a book, because it is difficult to know if the body is positioned correctly for each asana.

Relaxation

Apart from the problems of daily life, many other factors can cause stress and tension. Once the cause of the stress has been remedied, then the tension is released. If you feel under stress, try working with the visualisation for stress in Chapter 7. Tension in the physical body interferes with the functioning of all its systems, which can lead to complaints such as asthma, headaches, constipation, palpitations, heart problems and stomach ulcers. If you have lived with tension for many years, it will take time and practice to remedy this.

Firstly you have to develop awareness of it and then gradually learn to release it. Many people live in a state of tension for the best part of their lives without realising that they are tense. If you have suffered from tension over a period of years, it is not going to vanish miraculously overnight. But if the exercises and the visualisations are worked with regularly, in conjunction with periods of relaxation, then the mind and body will start to relax, health will improve and a greater sense of well-being will follow.

EXERCISE: SIMPLE RELAXATION TO START YOUR YOGA SESSION

☆ Lie on your back on the floor. Make sure that your body is straight and your chin tucked in. This allows the cervical spine to be stretched. Your legs should be slightly apart with your hands by your sides, palms facing upwards. If you suffer back problems, support the lower half of your legs from the knees down to your feet, either on a large cushion or over the seat of a chair. This reduces any tension in the spine.

☆ Start by relaxing your mind. Look at your thoughts as they pass through your mind. Visualise them as beautiful multi-coloured bubbles that float into the atmosphere and gently disperse. When your mind is relaxed, bring your concentration into your physical body. Starting with your feet, mentally feel each part of your body, and where you experience tension, gently allow yourself to release it. You might find it helpful to visualise these areas flooded with calming blue rays. When you have released as much tension from your body as you can, spend a few moments reflecting upon the state of relaxation you have achieved.

☆ On your next inhalation, raise your arms over your head, stretching the whole body. Exhaling, bring your arms back to your sides. Repeat this twice more before gently rolling over on to your side and sitting up in readiness to work with the asanas.

EXERCISE: *BADDHA KONASANA* (BASE CHAKRA – *MULADHARA* – RED)

The meaning of 'Baddha' is 'caught' or 'restrained' and the translation of 'kona' is an angle. This is a posture that one frequently sees Indian cobblers sitting in.

☆ Sit on the floor with your legs stretched out in front. Make sure that your spine is straight with your head correctly aligned to your body.

☆ Bend your knees and bring your feet close to the trunk of the body. Bring the soles of the feet together, holding the feet near the toes. Check to make sure that your spine is still straight. If you find that you have gone into a round shoulder posture, sit against a wall with a small cushion in the small of your back.

☆ Keeping the outer sides of both feet on the floor, bring the heels as close to the perineum as possible. Eventually, the heels should be in contact with this part of the body.

☆ Interlock the fingers and grip the feet firmly. Exhaling, gently lower the knees to the floor. If the inner thigh muscles and knee muscles are tight, you may only be able to lower the legs a few inches but, with practice, you should eventually be able to lower the knees to the floor. Hold the posture for as long as possible.

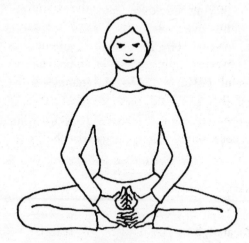

Baddha Konasana

☆ While holding the posture, bring your awareness to the Base chakra. With each inhalation, visualise a pure clear red coming from the earth, through your feet, up both your legs into this chakra. Feel the heaviness of this chakra, the heaviness that earths you to this planet. With each exhalation picture this clear red radiating from the chakra, into the lower part of your aura, down both your legs and back to the earth, creating a circuit of vibrant red energy. If your mind starts to wander, bring it back to the Base chakra and the visualisation.

☆ When you start to tire, release your feet, straighten your legs and relax for a few moments. During this time of relaxation, feel into your body for any changes that may have occurred. You can continue to visualise the Base chakra glowing with a vibrant red energy.

The Base chakra is the first chakra that deals with our survival instinct. It works with the reproductive organs, especially those of a male. Because the abdomen and the back are stimulated, the kidneys, prostate and bladder are kept healthy. This posture has a beneficial effect upon the ovaries, helps irregular menstruation and is a wonderful posture during pregnancy. It has been advocated that pregnant women who sit regularly in this posture will have an easier delivery and be free from varicose veins. This posture also helps to relieve sciatica.

EXERCISE: *PADANGUSTHASANA* (SACRAL CHAKRA – *SWADISTHANA* – ORANGE)

'Pada' means 'foot'. 'Angustha' is translated as 'big toe'.

☆ Begin in standing posture, checking to ensure that your spine is straight. Place your feet slightly apart so that each foot is in line with the hip. The feet should be parallel and the toes of the left and right foot in line.

☆ Inhale deeply, then on the exhalation bend the trunk of the body forward from the hips, keeping the spine straight and the knees locked, and hold the big toes with the hands. If you are unable to reach your toes, hold your legs. While holding this position, inhale, then on the next exhalation continue to lower the trunk of the body on to the legs.

☆ While holding this posture, bring your concentration into the Sacral chakra. On each inhalation, visualise a shaft of clear orange light rising from the earth, through

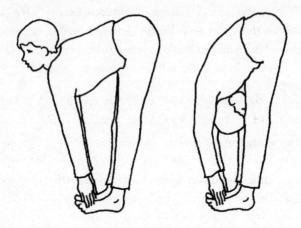

Padangusthasana

your feet, up your legs and into this centre. On the exhalation, allow this colour to radiate into your aura and back into the earth.

☆ When you feel that you can no longer hold the posture, inhale and raise your body back to standing posture. Relax for a moment and reflect on what you may have experienced.

This chakra is connected with our sexuality and our attitude towards it. If we are frigid or have sexual hangups, this centre becomes blocked. Working with this asana, the Sacral chakra and the colour orange will help to release negative sexual attitudes, enabling a full acceptance of life.

Physically, this posture works on the adrenal glands and the reproductive system, especially in women. It helps to eliminate constipation, indigestion and flatulence, makes the muscles of the back supple and stimulates the spinal nerves. It increases the flow of blood to the face and head. Anyone suffering from sciatica or serious back ailments should avoid doing this posture until their condition improves.

EXERCISE: *BHUJANGASANA* (SOLAR PLEXUS CHAKRA – *MANIPURA* – YELLOW)

'Bhujanga' means 'cobra'.

☆ Start this posture by lying face down with your chin resting on the floor. Place your hands by your chest with the fingers pointing towards the head.

☆ On your next inhalation, press down with your hands and lift the trunk of the body off the floor, making sure that you keep the pubis in contact with the floor and your legs straight. Take your shoulders down and back and keep your head in line with your spine. If you suffer from back problems, keep your forearms in contact with the floor and raise the trunk of your body from this position.

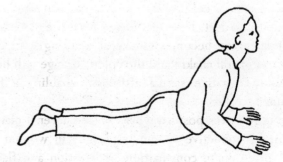

Bhujangasana

☆ While holding the posture, bring your concentration into the Solar Plexus chakra. On each inhalation, visualise a clear shaft of yellow light coming from the earth, through your feet, up your legs and into the chakra. On each exhalation imagine this colour radiating out into your aura and back down to the earth.

☆ When you start to tire, release the posture and lie face down on the floor in a relaxing position. Take note of any changes that may have taken place, physically, emotionally and mentally.

The element associated with this centre is fire, the fire of purification. The centre is also connected to the sun and yellow, this chakra's dominant colour being the one closest to sunlight. Only after we have burned away the dross in our lives are we able to experience the radiant beauty of our inner spiritual light. To do this, we have to work with and master the lessons that the three lower chakras teach. Only then are we able to experience the warmth and healing power of the spiritual light that resides in each living being. In the Dhammapada we find written:

If you find a man who is constant, awake to the
    inner light,
learned, long suffering, endowed with devotion, a
    noble man,
follow this good and great man even as the moon
    follows the path of the stars.

The cobra posture rejuvenates the spine and is beneficial for stiff backs, lumbago and sciatica. It tones the ovaries and uterus and helps to relieve disorders such as leucorrhea, dysmenorrhea and amenorrhea. It works on the kidneys and bladder and is good for alleviating water retention. It stimulates the appetite and eliminates constipation. This posture should not be practised by people suffering from stomach ulcers or a hernia.

EXERCISE: *UTTIHITA TRIKONASANA* (HEART CHAKRA – *ANAHATA* – GREEN)

'Uttihita' means 'stretched' and 'trikona' means 'triangle'.

☆ Start this asana in a standing posture, checking that your spine is straight. Extend the legs sideways three to three and a half feet. Turn the right foot sideways 90 degrees clockwise and the left foot slightly to the right. Contract the thigh muscles and tighten the knees. Raise your arms sideways in line with the shoulders, palms facing down.

☆ Inhale. On the next exhalation bend the trunk of the body to the right, allowing the right hand to hold the ankle.

☆ Raise the left arm upwards to form a line with the right shoulder. The backs of the legs, the back and the hips should be in line. Look up at the left hand. To check if you are in the correct position, this posture can be practised against a wall and your back should be against the wall when fully extended into the posture. If you find it difficult to reach your ankle, hold any part of your leg that allows the body to assume the correct position. If you are supple, you can extend your hand on to the floor.

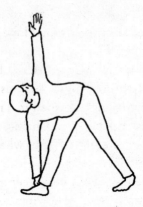

Uttihita Trikonasana

☆ While holding this posture, bring your awareness into the Heart chakra. With each inhalation, imagine a ray of clear green light entering this centre horizontally. With each exhalation, allow the colour to ray out into your aura.

☆ When you are ready, inhale and raise the trunk of the body. Now turn the left foot sideways 90 degrees anticlockwise and the right foot slightly to the left and repeat the posture again with the other side of your body, allowing your concentration to be centred on the Heart chakra. This time imagine a very pale pink rose bud with pale green leaves planted into your heart centre. Each time you practise this posture, picture yourself watering this bud watching as it slowly opens to full bloom.

☆ When you start to tire, bring the body back to standing posture and relax for a few moments, reflecting on what this chakra says to you. Try to find the imbalances in all aspects of your life and think of ways in which these can be rectified. Think of those that you do not

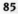

feel very charitable towards and try to send them the wonderful pink ray of unconditional love.

The Heart chakra is the centre of balance, lying midway between the three lower chakras and the three higher chakras. The triangle formed in Trikonasana can represent the three aspects of our being, namely body, mind and spirit, reminding us that when these three aspects are brought into balance we can become integrated into wholeness. The heart centre is also the centre of unconditional love. The vibrational frequency of this love empowers us to achieve harmony and balance.

This posture stimulates the nervous system and relieves nervous depression. It stimulates the appetite, improves digestion and helps to relieve constipation. It massages the spinal nerves, muscles of the lower back and the abdominal organs.

EXERCISE: *USTRASANA* (THROAT CHAKRA – *VISHUDDHA* – BLUE)

'Ustra' is translated as 'camel'.

☆ Start this posture in a kneeling position with your knees slightly apart.

☆ On the next exhalation, arch your back, take your hands back and place them on your heels. Stretch the neck backward letting the body weight rest on the arms. If you are unable to touch your feet, place cushions on your legs to the height required. As your back becomes more supple, reduce the number of cushions. In this posture it is important that the hips are kept in

line with the knees. One way of testing this is to practise the posture kneeling in front of a wall. When you
extend back to touch your feet, your thighs should not
lose contact with the wall.

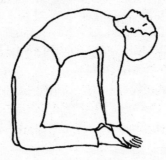

Ustrasana

☆ While holding this posture, breathe in a shaft of clear
blue light through the top of your head into the Throat
chakra. On the exhalation envisage this colour flowing
into your aura and back up towards the heavens. With
each in and out breath, allow this colour to instil into
you a wonderful sense of peace and relaxation. Try to
feel for any stagnation of energy that may be present in
this chakra. If you detect any, ask your higher self why
it is present and how you can work to remove it.

☆ When you are ready, release the posture, sit back on
your heels and relax for a few minutes. During this time
of relaxation turn your attention inwards to ascertain
what this posture has taught you.

The Throat chakra is also the centre of higher
creativity, of the spoken word and of sound. In many
people, this centre is blocked through their inability to

express their own truth and to follow the path that is right for them.

This asana is beneficial for the digestive, excretory and reproductive systems. It stretches the stomach and intestines, eliminating constipation. It helps to relieve backache and lumbago.

EXERCISE: *ARDHA MATSYENDRASANA* (BROW CHAKRA – *AJNA* – INDIGO)

This is translated as 'half abdominal twist'.

☆ Start by sitting on the floor, with the legs straight in front of the body.

☆ Bend the right leg and take it over the left leg, placing the sole of the foot on the floor by the left knee.

☆ Bend the left knee, placing the heel of the foot by the right buttock.

☆ Turn the trunk of the body to the right, placing the right hand on the floor, behind the body, with the fingers pointing away from the body. Make sure that both buttocks are kept in contact with the floor. On the next exhalation, turn the trunk of the body as far to the right as is possible, turning your head to look over the right shoulder. Hold for as long as possible.

☆ While holding this posture, bring your concentration into the Brow chakra. On each inhalation, envisage a ray of deep indigo coming through the top of your head and into the Brow chakra. On each exhalation see this colour radiate out into your aura to flow back to the universe.

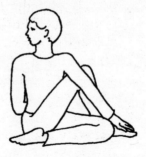

Ardha Matsyendrasana

☆ When the body starts to tire, change the legs over and repeat on the other side. After releasing the posture, relax for a few moments. Reflect on what you have experienced. Also look within yourself to try to discover how much space you have allowed yourself for your own spiritual development. Do you find it frightening to be in total silence? If so, why? If we are afraid of silence it can be an indication that we are trying to run away from something that we need to face. Remember, only through truth can we cross the bridge that leads to the higher realms of consciousness.

This chakra is often referred to as the third eye, the eye of wisdom. It is the place where one can listen to the higher self, the intuition. The colour indigo is sometimes referred to as the colour of the 'vaults of heaven', the colour of stillness and space. In order to be able to listen and to learn to trust our intuition, we need to create for ourselves physical, emotional and mental space. This practice will ultimately lead us to find our own inner space, where ultimate peace, joy, security and love dwell. Yoga philosophy tells us that next to the heart centre is a small chamber. On entering it we find an altar bedecked with many precious jewels and upon the altar resides the true self.

On a physical level, this posture makes the back muscles supple and tones the spinal nerves. It massages the abdominal organs, removing digestive ailments. It works on the adrenal glands and the pancreas and helps to relieve lumbago and muscular rheumatism.

EXERCISE: *PRASARITA PADOTTANASANA* (CROWN CHAKRA – *SAHASRARA* – VIOLET)

This is translated as 'expanded foot posture'.

☆ Start this asana in a standing posture. Walk the feet sideways until they are three to four feet apart.

☆ On the next exhalation, bend from the hips, making sure that the spine is kept straight, and place both hands on the floor, fingers facing forward. If your body is stiff, preventing you from reaching all the way down, arrange a pile of books on the floor in front of you to put your hands on.

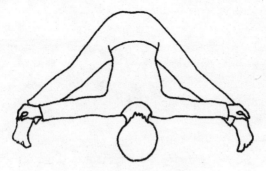

Prasarita Padottanasana

☆ Slowly walk the hands backwards until they are in

line with the feet. At the same time, extend the trunk of the body until the head rests on the floor.

☆ When you have achieved this position, you can hold the left ankle with your left hand and your right ankle with your right hand.

☆ Bring your awareness into the Crown chakra. With each inhalation, visualise a violet beam of light entering this centre and radiating into the aura. Look to the centre of this beam of violet light and try to find the pure white ray of light that is always present. This is the light which connects us to the spiritual world.

The Crown chakra is the centre of pure consciousness. It awakens when we have brought all aspects of our life into the balance of polarity. When this has been achieved, we have reached the goal of many lifetimes; we have become one with that divine spark, the light that dwells in all living things. Different religions give different names to this state. In yoga it is the attainment of the last step – samadhi or enlightenment.

This posture brings a rich supply of blood to the brain. It works on the inner thighs and hamstring muscles. It removes stiffness from the shoulders and fully opens the chest. This posture should not be done by persons suffering high blood pressure.

☆ When you have finished your yoga session, lie on the floor and cover yourself with a blanket. Spend the next 15 to 20 minutes in relaxation. While relaxing, mentally go over your body, noting any changes. Consider each chakra, starting from the base, and look once more at their spiritual attributes and the brilliance of the colour that radiates from them. Try to tune into your own intuition and listen to what it is trying to tell you. Ask any questions that you are seeking the answers to.

☆ When you feel ready, bring your arms over your head, stretching the whole body. Gently lower your arms to your sides, roll over on to your left-hand side and sit up.

6

Colour Breathing: Pranayama

Pranayama is a prayer, not mere physical exercise.

B.K.S. Iyengar

Another way of working with colour is with the breath. The air that we breathe contains prana derived from the sun (see page 31). Prana contains the seven spectral colours, so the very act of breathing feeds our aura and physical body with the vibrational energies of the colours needed to sustain life. Consciously visualising specific colours when inhaling and directing these to the parts of our body where we feel they are needed increases the intake of energy afforded by these colours to those specific body areas. Prana is a vital force that permeates our mind, body and spirit, giving us not only our existence but also the feeling for and enjoyment of life.

The Air We Breathe

Unfortunately, the air that we breathe today is no longer pure but polluted with dust from heavy industry and emissions from car exhausts, which both deplete the air of prana, oxygen and negative ions, substances vital to our well-being. The atmosphere in which we live contains both negative and positive ions, electrically charged atoms which give life to the cellular structure of plants, animals and humans. Negative ions, minute packets of very active electrical energy in an almost pure state, are usually formed of several oxygen or nitrogen atoms. Positive ions are much larger and slower and have the ability to trap negative ions, causing an overproduction of positive ones, as when the air is polluted with dust, smoke or fog and the conductivity of the air is diminished. Negative ions help the passage of oxygen through cell membranes by increasing the pressure of oxygen in the air cells of the lungs and decreasing the carbon dioxide, thus making the absorption of oxygen by the blood easier. Positive ions have the reverse effect. For this reason, it is essential to find a place to work with the breathing exercises that has little or no pollution. If you live in a large city, try to find an open space, such as a park, where there is minimal traffic.

It is a known medical fact that the majority of the population use only one-third of their lungs' capacity. Learning to increase this capacity results in a greater intake of prana, but this should be done gradually over a period of time. If performed too suddenly the lungs could loose some of their elasticity. Although breathing is a natural occurrence, an abrupt change in the way we breathe can have other detrimental effects. When we start to increase the length of our inhalation and exhalation, we absorb more oxygen than the body is used to, which can result in hyperventilation, producing giddiness. Another occurrence can be an accumulation of carbon dioxide in the lungs, creating breathlessness. When working with the breathing techniques given, resume normal breathing immediately if either of these symptoms should occur.

Working with these exercises with awareness helps us to learn to listen to our body – something that very few people do. When we are able to listen to our body, it will tell us the type of food it requires, when it needs to rest or be active and the colours it requires to help maintain optimum health. Working in this way teaches us to become the master of ourself.

When you start to work with breathing exercises it is important that you do not retain the breath for more than a count of two. Retention of the breath is a way in which energy is moved and directed in the body. To do this effectively, the body has to be strong. If this is your first introduction to pranayama, restrict your practice session to a maximum of 15 minutes. It is advisable to practise all breathing exercises in the morning, preferably in the open air, but if this is not possible in a well-ventilated room. Practising in the evening could energise the body, making sleep difficult. If you smoke cigarettes, refrain from this for at least one hour prior to working with these exercises. Smoking has an adverse effect on the respiratory system, circulatory system and adrenal glands.

EXERCISE: PRACTISING SLOW INHALATION AND EXHALATION

☆ In a well-ventilated room, sit in a position that is comfortable but enables your spine to be straight, with your shoulders down and back and your chest open. This allows space for the expansion of the lungs and for the diaphragm to extend into the abdominal cavity during inhalation, a posture that should be adopted for all breathing exercises. Always breathe through your nose to ensure that the air is the correct temperature, free from dust and for the the maximum absorption of prana.

☆ Bring your awareness to the tip of your nose. Slowly inhale to a count of five. Feel the air entering your nose and travelling through your pharynx, trachea, bronchial tubes and into your lungs.

☆ Hold for a count of two, before slowly exhaling to five. As you exhale, be aware of the change in temperature of the exhaled air as it passes out through your nose.

☆ Repeat for five to ten minutes making sure that the inhalation is kept the same length as the exhalation. If you find that you become breathless counting to five, reduce the count to four or three. If you find the count too short, then increase it.

On completing this exercise, your metabolism should have slowed down and you should be experiencing a sense of peace and relaxation. These feelings will increase with practice.

Introducing Colour

☆ Work either with the colour you intuitively feel you need or one selected from your bag of ribbons. Like the first exercise, it is important to make your inhalation the same length as your exhalation.

☆ Sitting quietly, look at the colour of your chosen ribbon. Contemplate its meaning for you. If it helps, reread Chapter 4 before you start the exercise.

☆ When you feel ready, close your eyes and visualise your chosen colour. It may help if you visualise something in nature that radiates the same colour. On your next inhalation, breathe the colour in through your nose and, as you exhale, visualise the colour penetrating and saturating every part of yourself, from your feet to your head.

☆ Continue to work in this way for five to ten minutes. At the end of this time, sit quietly for a few moments pondering any changes that may have occurred in either your body or the way you feel.

EXERCISE: BALANCING THE CHAKRAS WITH COLOUR

When working with this exercise, the earth colours red, orange and yellow are visualised entering the body through the feet; green penetrates the heart chakra horizontally; and blue, indigo and violet enter through the head. Repeat each stage three to six times.

☆ Sitting quietly, take a few slow breaths to quieten your mind and relax your body before starting the exercise.

☆ When you feel ready, on your next inhalation visualise the bright, clear red of a rose coming from the earth, into your feet and legs and being absorbed into the Base chakra. As you breathe out, watch the colour flowing from the chakra into your aura, down your legs and back to the earth.

☆ Change the colour to a bright clear orange, the colour of marigolds. On your next inhalation, bring this colour from the earth into your feet and legs to the Sacral chakra. When you sense that this chakra is full with colour, exhale, picturing the colour spinning from the chakra, into your aura and back to the earth.

☆ On your next inhalation, visualise the bright clear yellow displayed on the outer petals of daffodils, rising from the earth, through your feet and up into the Solar Plexus chakra. Working with this centre, you watch the colour yellow infusing it with the warmth and radiance of the sun. As you breathe out, these rays of light penetrate and spread throughout your aura, generating warmth and energy to your physical body.

☆ Shift your concentration to your Heart chakra. Contemplate the warmth of a sunny spring day, encouraging the buds on the trees to open and bring forth their newly formed green leaves. With each inhalation, fill your Heart chakra with this colour; with each exhalation observe the colour flowing through the small branchlike channels found in the etheric part of your aura, clearing away any stagnant energy encountered in its path. As you work with this colour, try to experience the calmness and sense of balance that it brings you.

☆ Raising your awareness to the Throat chakra, imagine yourself sitting beneath a clear, blue summer sky. As you inhale and bring this colour through the top of your head and into this chakra, it expands and with each exhalation pushes rays of blue light into your aura. This causes your aura to widen and to unite itself and you with the infinite space of the sky. The feeling this gives you is one of indescribable joy and peace.

☆ Moving to the Brow chakra, change the blue of the summer sky into the deep indigo of night. As you breathe this colour into your Brow chakra, the sense of limitless space around you increases and becomes filled with a deep, breathless silence. Try to take this silence and space inside of yourself. Practice will eventually enable you to find your own inner space, containing all that you could possibly wish for.

☆ With the sense of peace, silence and space surrounding you, lift your awareness to the Crown chakra. As you inhale, visualise a deep violet light filling this centre. Exhaling, breathe this colour into your aura and ask that it may teach you to love every aspect of yourself, no matter how imperfect you think these may be. In time you will grow to unconditionally love not only yourself but all things surrounding you.

☆ At the end of this exercise, sit quietly for a few minutes, reflecting your experiences. Remember: the more you practise, the greater the benefits.

Meridians

Another way of breathing colour into yourself is through the governing and conception meridians, which go to make up the 14 bilateral meridians found in the human body. Bilateral means that the meridians, excluding the governing and conception ones, are found on both the right and left side of the body.

The governing meridian acts as a kind of environmental gauge and is strongly affected by changes in pressure, humidity and temperature. It is adversely affected by chocolate and chemicals. When this meridian is weak, fatigue and lack of will surface. The conception meridian is responsible for the electric charge and current throughout the body. Depressed people and those who cannot see or meet their goals in life will have a low current flowing through this meridian. Conversely, a person who is a high achiever will have the conception meridian highly charged.

The governing meridian runs from the perineum up the back, in line with the spine, up the back of the head, across the crown and down the forehead, terminating on the hard palate behind the two front teeth. The conception meridian comes from the perineum up the centre of the front of the body and through the neck, terminating on the tip of the tongue. In order to create a circuit of energy with these two meridians, the tip of the tongue, where the conception meridian terminates, must be placed at the termination point of the governing meridian, on the hard palate behind the two front teeth.

Exercise: Working the Meridians Using Colour

☆ Sitting quietly, select the colour that you feel you need, either intuitively or through your bag of ribbons. Try to ascertain if you need this colour physically, mentally, emotionally or spiritually.

☆ With a relaxed body and quiet mind, bring your concentration to the perineum. On your next inhalation visualise your chosen colour travelling from the perineum up the governing meridian to its point of termination, behind the two front teeth.

☆ Making sure that the tip of your tongue is resting

behind your two front teeth, exhale, visualising the colour entering the tip of your tongue and flowing down the conception meridian, back to the perineum.

☆ Continue to bring the colour into the governing meridian with each inhalation and down the conception meridian with each exhalation, remembering to keep your tongue in contact with the governing meridian's termination point. Work with this exercise for five to ten minutes, picturing yourself slowly becoming cocooned in a brilliant orb of your chosen colour. When you have completed the exercise, spend a few moments reflecting its effect upon you.

EXERCISE: ABSORBING ALL SEVEN COLOURS

☆ Sitting quietly, bring your concentration to the crown of your head. As you inhale, imagine a shaft of white light entering through the Crown chakra, passing through your body and out of your feet.

☆ As this light travels through each of your chakras, the chakra takes from the light the colour it vibrates to. The Crown chakra absorbs the violet, the Brow absorbs indigo, the Throat absorbs blue, the Heart absorbs green, the Solar Plexus absorbs yellow, the Sacral absorbs orange and the Base chakra absorbs red. Continue to work with this exercise until you feel all your body resonating to the energy given by light.

7

Colour Visualisations and Meditations

A meditative mind is silent. It is not the silence of a still evening; it is the silence when thought – with all its images, its words and perceptions – has entirely ceased. The meditative mind is the religious mind – the religion that is not touched by the church, the temples or by chants.

The religious mind is the explosion of love. It is this love that knows no separation. To it, far is near. It is not the one or the many, but rather that state of love in which all division ceases. Like beauty, it is not of the measure of words. From the silence alone the meditative mind acts.

J. Krishnamurti

Meditation is increasingly popular. I hear people talking about the meditation classes they are attending, how often and when they practise, which technique they are working with. But, when asked why they are pursuing this particular path, the answers given are usually vague and based on their belief that it helps them to relax. Meditation does aid relaxation, but its true purpose goes far beyond this.

Finding the True Self

The teaching behind all religions and esoteric paths is to discover our true self – who we really are. The name given to us, our address or social activities are all things *about* us. If they were removed and there was no external factor by which to describe ourselves, then who would we be? 'Know thyself' is the classical philosophical advice offered by both Eastern and Western masters. But who or what is this 'self' and how do we go about finding it?

In order to find 'self' and the place where it dwells, we first have to learn to quieten and transcend our rational, thinking mind. This is far from easy and takes both patience and practice. We also have to learn how to create within and around ourselves a state of silence. This for many is an alien state, which can create feelings of fear. In the modern world noise has become the norm, constantly surrounding us at both home and work, so learning to work with silence is difficult. Once this has been achieved, the slightest noise becomes a form of pollution. Meditation is one method to help us to quieten and transcend our rational, thinking mind to achieve the state of consciousness that allows us to realise our true 'self'.

Meditation can take many forms, such as transcendental meditation, working with geometric form (yantras or mandalas), using sound (mantras), working with the breath (pranayama) and using visualisation. For those who have had no previous experience with meditation, I feel that working with visualisation is the easiest way to start. This chapter provides meditations that work with both colour and visualisation so that you can experience for yourself their uniqueness and power. When you have worked with these, you might like to create your own or explore some of the other techniques listed above.

When starting to work with meditation, it is advisable to practise in a place that is free from noise and distractions. It is recommended that you always practise in the same place, because over a period of time you will build up positive vibrations that will help you attain a meditative state more quickly. Objects such as crystals, chimes, coloured scarves and flowers can be placed around your space and candles and incense can be burned if you find it helpful. If this is the first time that you have worked with meditation, it is important to practise initially for 20 minutes on a regular daily basis and preferably at the same time each day. This creates a discipline that will help you. It is so easy to start the day with good intentions and end the day without fulfilling them.

Another important point to remember is that each practice session is a unique and complete experience. Therefore, don't try to recapture the glorious and fulfilling moments that you will from time to time experience. This serves no purpose, because the very act of trying stands in the way. There will also be many times, especially in the beginning, when you spend the whole practice session trying to focus your mind. Don't give up. This happens to everyone.

When you have found a suitable place to practise, adopt a sitting posture that is comfortable and allows your spine to be upright. If you choose to sit on a chair, place both feet on the floor and both hands on your thighs, palms facing down. If you sit on the floor, sit with your back against a wall, with a small cushion placed in the small of your back. Start each session by concentrating on your breath, making your inhalations the same length as your exhalations. With each exhalation, breathe out any tension you may be feeling. At the end of each session, it is important to remember to close down your chakras. These are your doors to higher consciousness and when meditating they open more fully. The easiest way to close them is to visualise each centre as an open flower. Starting at the Crown chakra and working down to the Base, visualise each flower closing back to a bud. You might then like to visualise yourself inside an orb of golden protective light.

MEDITATIONS USING COLOUR WITH VISUALISATION

Quietening the Mind in Preparation for Visualisation

☆ Sitting in your chosen place, bring your concentration into your breath, making your inhalation the same length as your exhalation. When you feel your body start to relax, shift your awareness to your thoughts. Try to be an onlooker, impartial to the constant stream of thoughts passing through your mind. Start to visualise these thoughts as beautiful multi-coloured bubbles that float into the atmosphere and melt, leaving your mind at peace and focused to work with your chosen visualisation.

EXERCISE: SILENCE

☆ Imagine yourself lying in a grassy field beneath a clear blue sky. As you travel into its depths, the blue gradually changes into a deep indigo, which creates a vault of space and silence. Rest for a few moments to listen to and experience this grand silence. If you experience fear, try asking yourself the reason why. Being constantly surrounded by the noise pollution ever present on earth, we can forget what it is like to be silent, so this initially can make silence feel uncomfortable. But this silence is needed to enable you to look into all aspects of yourself.

☆ Looking back to earth, you see it bathed in golds and yellows created from the sun's light. Yellow is the colour that permits us to stand back and review our life, and gold gives us the wisdom to change aspects of our life to allow for new growth and understanding.

☆ As you survey this scene, do you feel that there are things that you need to change or to let go of so that you may walk forward in life? If so, ask that you may be given the wisdom to undertake these changes wisely.

☆ Stay for a while, surrounded by the silence and space that indigo allows and try to listen to your inner voice of wisdom.

EXERCISE: HARDNESS AND BITTERNESS

☆ It is winter, and you are looking out of the window of a cottage situated in the middle of the countryside. Newly fallen snow has hardened with the extreme coldness of the past night. Each tiny flake has become a crystal of frozen water, displaying its own unique pattern. As the new day dawns and the sun makes its way across a cloudless sky, each tiny water crystal, as it becomes bathed in the warmth of the sun, starts to melt, releasing its inner multi-coloured light, which plays across the vast expanse of white.

☆ As you contemplate this scene, look to yourself. Do

you have any hardness that has accumulated through hatred, anger, resentment or bitterness? If you have and you don't resolve these feelings then, like the frozen water crystals, your own inner light will not be able to shine forth.

☆ Bringing your concentration to your Solar Plexus chakra, visualise this as a golden sun whose beams of light reach into every aspect of your being, melting any negativity, bitterness or hardness that you may be harbouring. As these feelings dissolve in the warmth of the sun's light, see the void they leave behind being filled with your own inner light, which radiates from your heart centre to flood you and the space where you are sitting.

EXERCISE: STEADFASTNESS OF SPIRIT

☆ Envisage yourself sitting secure and warm in a small secluded cave set in the cliffs above a pale yellow sandy beach. A storm brews outside, sending the incoming waves rolling over the sands and hurtling into the cliffs. The white froth formed on the top of the waves hits the cliffs with a loud explosion, then shatters and falls back into the receding water. The wind howls, chasing the black and grey clouds, which shed a torrent of rain as they race across the sky.

☆ Unexpectedly, a break appears in the clouds and the golden rays of the sun appear, spreading an arc of rainbow-coloured light across the sky.

☆ Each of us has a secure and sheltered cave within, frequently referred to as our inner space. Once we have discovered and learned to rest in this space, we can always stand strong, untroubled and secure, no matter how fierce the storms of life. When we are able to function from our inner space we are able to direct our own inner light into those places where there is darkness, war, hatred and envy. Look to this place so that you may rest serene and strong amidst life's troubled waters.

EXERCISE: FINDING YOUR OWN INNER SPACE

☆ Sitting quietly, bring your concentration to your Heart chakra. Visualise this as a pulsating circle of pale green light. With each exhalation, imagine this circle growing in size, until it takes the shape of a large circular room, with you sitting inside.

☆ Looking around, you note that the inside of the room is filled with a soft, white light. At its centre lies a water pool surrounded by crystals and precious stones displaying varied hues of red, orange, yellow, green, turquoise, blue and violet. Each stone penetrates the light with its own colour hue and special energy. Listening carefully, you start to hear the soft pure sound that each stone and crystal is vibrating to, each one blending with all others to create a perfect harmonious symphony. In this place you find peace, relaxation and detachment from all external problems and pressures, enabling you to see them in a new light. You feel empowered and the master of your own life and find the security, strength and truth that can never be shaken by outward things.

☆ Whenever you feel afraid, or threatened by outer

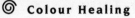

circumstances, quietly return to this special place to find what you need to allow you to stand firm and secure.

EXERCISE: TENSION

Tension affects every system in our physical body and can cause headaches, constipation, stiffness and stomach ulcers. If we wish to be well and healthy, we have to learn to eliminate tension and stress from our lives.

☆ Imagine yourself sitting in front of a small deep blue sapphire stone. As you gaze at this stone visualise it growing into the size of a small room.

☆ Standing up and walking round this now huge crystal you find a door, which you open and walk through into a circular crystal room filled with soft blue light. Upon the floor is a deep pile white carpet upon which are scattered white cushions of all shapes and sizes. In the centre of the room a small fountain plays.

☆ Selecting some of the cushions, lie down on the carpet, placing the cushions beneath your head and knees for comfort. As your body starts to relax, try to locate any areas of tension. Visualise the blue rays of light flooding these areas, gently releasing the tension to allow your muscles to become soft and pliable and all systems of your physical body to function more efficiently. When you feel that you have released your tension, try to examine and resolve the cause of it. This may initially prove difficult, especially if it involves change, which in its many forms is never easy but can give us a wonderful opportunity for growth and learning. All that stress and tension will do is to eventually make us ill. Quietly relaxing, bring your attention to the sound of the water, allowing its gentle rhythm to take you into sleep.

EXERCISE: WORKING WITH DEPRESSION

☆ Sitting in a quiet, peaceful place, start this visualisation with a few deep inhalations and exhalations to quieten your mind and relax your body.

☆ When you feel ready, imagine yourself sitting in the countryside just before the break of dawn. The sky is filled with dark rain clouds, cloaking you and the landscape with a thick, dark blanket, obliterating the small amount of light normally offered by the stars and moon.

☆ While sitting in this state of heaviness and darkness, unable to see anything around you, dawn starts to break, piercing the dark clouds with a single ray of golden orange light. This colour floods the space where you sit. As it slowly starts to disperse your own dark clouds of depression you are able to look at yourself and the way you feel. Finally the sun, in its full glory, appears over the horizon, transforming the sky into a blaze of orange and red light, filling the atmosphere with these vibrant colours and dissolving what remains of your own cloud of darkness. Lying down in these glorious colours, you allow them to penetrate all parts of yourself. Breathing in the orange rays lifts your spirits and renews your energies, allowing you to see the path you should take. Stay with this scene until you feel ready to continue your day.

EXERCISE: DETOXIFICATION OF THE PHYSICAL BODY

The fast, chemically impregnated food of our present life-style can make our physical body toxic, depleting us of energy. One way of working with this problem is by changing our diet. For example, we could eat just fruit for breakfast, salad for lunch and vegetables with either lean meat or fish for our evening meal. Coffee and tea could be replaced with mineral water and herb teas. Initially this idea may appear uninteresting or prove difficult, but I can assure you it does become easier and more enjoyable once an increase in energy and a greater sense of well-being is experienced.

☆ Sitting in a comfortable and relaxed position, imagine yourself standing outside a circular building. Walking around the outside of this building you find the door, which you push open and walk through, into a circular room filled with streaming sunlight from the room's many windows. At the centre of the room a large fountain plays, flooded with lime green light from the central ceiling's stained glass.

☆ Approaching the fountain, place your hand into the warm water to feel the wonderful sensation of lightness and cleanliness this gives to it. Now step into the centre of the fountain, where the gentle fall of the water, impregnated with lime green, cleanses your aura of stagnated energy and helps to detoxify your physical body.

☆ When you feel refreshed and clean, step out from the fountain and sit for a while in the peaceful atmosphere afforded to this room to reflect upon yourself and your life-style.

EXERCISE: WORKING WITH THE DYING

To me, the act of dying is the laying down of the physical body, freeing the soul to return to its spiritual home. This, I feel, is a complete transformation and healing process but, for many people, death holds tremendous fear. If you know someone who is passing through death, holding them in your imagination in both colour and light aids this transformation.

☆ Sitting in a comfortable place, visualise the dying person lying at peace, free from pain and fear. Visualise angelic beings of light surrounding the bed, waiting to greet the soul as it leaves the body and escort it to its spiritual home. See the dying person surrounded by a very pale magenta light, helping them detach from the earthly realm and infusing them with unconditional love.

☆ Visualise the radiant soul of the person leaving their body to be met and taken into spirit by relatives and friends who have already passed over. Looking back at the vacated body, see this as an empty shell that you bless and thank for the life that it has sustained.

EXERCISE: CIRCLE OF LIGHT

☆ Sitting quietly, visualise yourself standing on the outer border of a large circle filled with colour and light. The place where you are standing is illuminated with a soft, clear red. Contemplate the effect that this colour has upon you. If you feel that you need this colour in any part of your body, absorb it with each inhalation into those parts until they become saturated with red light.

☆ Walking towards the centre of the circle, you move out of the red and into the orange ray. Feel the subtle differences produced by this colour's energy. If you feel the need to stay for a while wrapped in the energising, joyful and creative power that this colour brings, do so.

☆ Coming out of the orange, you walk into the yellow ray. This gives you the sensation of sitting beneath the warming rays of the sun. Imagine this colour entering your eyes to work with all your body systems in order that you may become strong and healthy for your chosen mission in life.

☆ Continuing your journey, you enter the green ray of light. This is reminiscent of walking through a thickly wooded forest in midsummer. The sun's rays, shining through the leafy arches, light the ground below with a soft translucent green, which helps to slow down your metabolism and aids your body to find its own state of equilibrium. Rest here for a while before moving on.

☆ As you move out from the green to the blue ray, the scene changes to a field carpeted with bluebells. This colour blesses you with peace and relaxation by helping to release tension in your body and mind.

☆ Nearing the circle's centre, you pass from the blue into the deep indigo of night. The contrast between the blue ray's energy and the energy of the indigo is dynamic. The silence and space with which you are now surrounded allows you time to reflect and heal any old, negative feelings of hurt that still lie buried within you. Visualise this colour penetrating and gently dissolving these feelings to allow you to appreciate and experience fully the next colour.

☆ Violet is the colour that stands next to the circle's centre. Walking into this colour is like walking into the centre of an amethyst crystal. Its rays permit you to be strong and to appreciate yourself for what you are. As human beings we are unique and carry within ourselves that primordial light out of which all things became manifest.

☆ Stepping out of the violet ray, we finally enter the centre of the circle, where we become immersed in its radiant white light, composed of all the spectral colours, which surround and interpenetrate us. If we are able to enter the heart, the centre of our own being, we will contact our own inner light, which has always been and will always be present. Once we have found this place, we are then able to radiate our light into those places where disease, darkness, war and hatred dwell.

EXERCISE: REALISATION

☆ Imagine a huge beech tree dressed in rich, shining autumnal colour. The warm russet and copper, the crimson and red, the gold and deep green are displayed in the delightful shapes of the tree's leaves. The whole majestic tree glistens as the light from the sun streams through small openings left by the intertwining branches.

☆ This scene teaches that each of us has to find our own small openings where our inner truth and light shines through. By practising colour meditations and developing colour awareness these small openings grow enabling greater light and understanding to come to and flow from us.

8

Mandalas

We have to try to reveal that Light which is hidden in us
   as a bud.
It must blossom like a flower. In all things everywhere, in
   all beings,
the Light is hidden, and it must be revealed.

Mother Meera

One of my favourite ways of working with colour is through
mandalas. For me, these create a wonderful media for self-
expression and self-revelation. At the end of a very busy day,
settling down with paints, crayons and paper to create and
colour these symbolic pictures establishes for me a wonderful
sense of peace and a state of relaxation. Working in this way
allows my brain to 'switch off', guaranteeing a restful night's
sleep.

The word 'mandala', comes from Sanskrit and means
'centre', 'circumference' or 'magic circle'. Mandalas are
created from two basic essentials, a circle and a centre point.
The circle represents eternity, because it has no beginning
and no ending. Magical rites throughout the ages have always

been performed within a circle, because it was – and still is – the belief that anything enacted within the circle is protected. The central point symbolises the sun, the Divine Light or sky door, which allows us access to our divine self.

There are many ways of using mandalas. Hindus, Tibetan Buddhists and Native Americans use them as an aid to healing. The psychologist Carl Gustav Jung, learned from his own inner turmoil that mandalas are a powerful tool for accessing the subconscious and unconscious minds. They are also tools for meditation, revealing and expanding the light that is within each of us. The mandalas in this chapter can help you to express yourself through colour and be an aid to meditation. Working in this way will help your awareness and appreciation of colour to grow.

The first mandala is based on the Platonic solids, a name given to the five three-dimensional solids considered to have special significance in the Platonic Schools of Greece and Alexandria.

In the explanation given for this mandala, the colours normally attributed to these solids have been given for your use and interest. The second and third mandalas are taken from rose windows, large circular windows, found in Romanesque and Gothic cathedrals, that are divided by elaborate tracery, with a central compartment from which other sections radiate. These divisions are filled with pieces of stained glass, often to powerful effect. When I was working in Switzerland, the grounds that housed the centre were I was teaching contained a church with a rose window. When the sun shone through this window it filled the church with streams of coloured light. Our group visited this church on several occasions, finding the spectacle a wonderful source of inspiration and joy. I hope that you also find inspiration and joy from working with the mandalas.

Before starting to work with the mandalas, it would be advisable to have them photocopied and enlarged. Take several photocopies of each, so that you can experiment with different colour combinations. It is amazing how different colours can provide completely different effects. Work with either paint or a good set of coloured pencils that contain a variety of shades that blend easily together. You can work each mandala, either with colours that you feel complement each other and enhance the symbolism or you can work with colours that you feel drawn towards.

When you have finished colouring your mandala, place it where you can comfortably see it. Read the interpretation to see if this speaks truth for you, then look at the colours you have used to see if they are telling you something about yourself. When you have done this, starting at the outer edge of the circle, slowly and gently allow your gaze to wander to the central point. Be open to feelings, ideas or insights that this may provoke. At the end of the exercise, sit quietly for a few moments to reflect on your experiences. If at first you have difficulty concentrating your mind, remember that this will improve with regular practice.

When you have worked with the mandalas, try creating your own. They do not have to be perfect or great works of art. The very act of creating them can be therapeutic. The only tools that you require are a compass, ruler, paper and pencils.

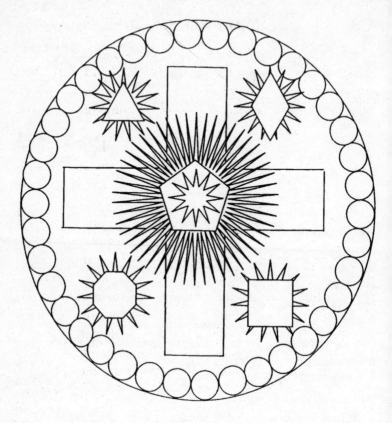

Mandala No. 1

Mandala No. 1

This mandala allows you to experiment with colour. The colour for the Platonic shapes, the rays of light behind these and the cross are described here. You may choose to use these colours or experiment with colours of your own choice.

The gold equal-limbed cross symbolises: the four corners of the earth – north, south, east and west; the four elements – earth, water, fire and air; and the four aspects of ourselves – body, mind, emotion and spirit.

At the lower right-hand corner lies the square or hexahedron. This relates to the element earth and is normally associated with the colour green. Moving in an anticlockwise direction, the next shape is the icosahedron. This is related to the element water and the colour blue. Moving across from the icosahedron we come to the tetrahedron, related to the element of fire and the colour red. Below the tetrahedron is the octahedron which is affiliated to the element air and the colour yellow. In the centre of the cross lies the dodecahedron radiating the colour violet and affiliated to the element of ether. Behind each of these solids (shown in two-dimensional form in this diagram) blaze rays of deep yellow light. The star in the centre of the dodecahedron shines with a golden orange light. The colours of the circles around the circumference of the mandala are for you to choose and colour in, before colouring the background the deep indigo of night.

This mandala speaks of balancing all aspects of ourself in order to reach the divine light within.

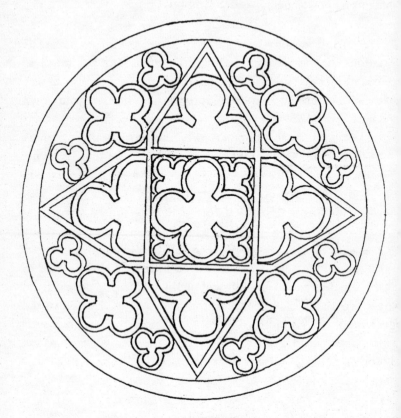

Mandala No. 2

Mandala No. 2

This mandala speaks about working to overcome duality in order to reach a state of wholeness. As you contemplate it you will notice that it embodies the numbers three and four. The outer part of the circle is divided into four sections, each containing three apertures. Within, there are four triangular shapes at whose centre lies a four-sided square containing a four-sided figure.

The number three invites us to contemplate the three aspects of ourselves – body, mind and spirit. Only when we have worked to integrate these are we able to reach a state of wholeness. This number also reminds us of the three stages of earthly existence – birth, life and death – and of the three virtues needed on our spiritual journey – truth, courage and compassion. Reflect for a while upon your own life, your failings and your achievements. Are you able to work with truth, exercise courage and show compassion? What are your thoughts on the last stages of life, namely death? Death is a topic that very few people choose to talk about, mainly because it is something they fear. But is death a process that takes us into a new phase of existence?

The square at the centre of the mandala is related to the earth. When we aspire to spiritual truths, we must make sure that we stay grounded by keeping our feet firmly on the earth. Only by doing this can we integrate our spiritual with our earthly life. This is important if we are to fulfil the mission that we came here to do.

The four-sided figure within the square represents our spiritual door. Four is the number of wholeness and completion. When we reach this state, we have completed our journey and become one with the Supreme Being.

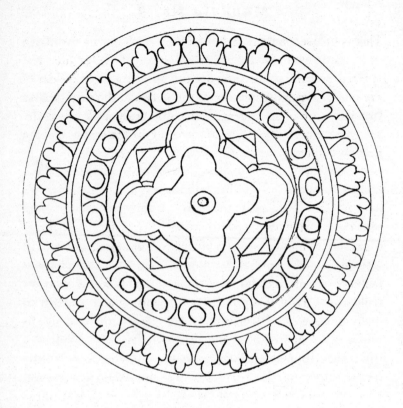

Mandala No. 3

Mandala No. 3

This is the second mandala based on a rose window. Each time I look at it, for me it resembles a pattern for life. The apertures forming the outer part of the circle remind me of the many barriers we put up against life and the many masks that we wear in an endeavour to hide the person we really are. The circular patterns that form the next part of the mandala resemble the layers of an onion and remind me of the layers formed around ourselves through conditioning and fear. Only when we gently peel away these layers can we see ourselves for what we are. Moving towards the centre we find the strength and stability of the earth, depicted in the square, and the four-sided figure representing wholeness.

Until we have worked with ourselves, acknowledging our faults and shortcomings, we cannot possibly know who we truly are. Part of this process is recognising and working to overcome the ego, because this can be destructive and give us a false sense of worth. Peeling away the layers that we have surrounded ourselves with can be painful, because it often exposes our vulnerability. But, if we can clothe ourselves in a beautiful rainbow of light, as we gently peel away these layers our vulnerability will be protected during the process of learning to truthfully accept ourselves for what we really are.

As you meditate on this mandala, try to feel the layers around yourself that need to be peeled away. Look at the many masks you wear and ask yourself why you need to use these. Learning to become yourself takes time, patience and a sense of humour. If we can learn to laugh at ourselves, it makes the whole process a lot easier.

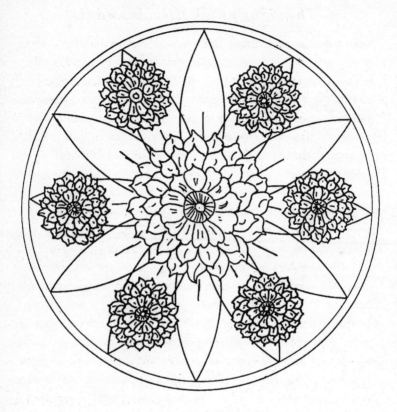

The Flower of Life

The Flower of Life Mandala

I can visualise each living thing as a flower in a different stage of growth. Some flowers have not yet come to bud, others still have their petals furled tightly around them, many are just starting to open and a few have reached the perfection and beauty of full blossom.

The six flowers around the circumference of this mandala represent the first six chakras, the doors that have to be gently opened before we can reach the Crown chakra of enlightenment. Each of these chakras has both negative and positive attributes and, when in a state of balance, they provide us with strong positive energy. But if they become over- or undercharged, their energy becomes negative. In the average person, the chakras are in a constant state of change, determined by that person's emotional and mental state.

When we strive to work with our own negativity, we start to see glimpses of the unlimited knowledge and beauty of the universe through the Crown chakra. As we open this centre, represented by the central flower on the mandala, we start to understand and work with cosmic law and to embrace unconditional love.

As you work with the Flower of Life, visualise and feel into your own chakras. On reaching the central flower, imagine a shaft of brilliant light entering the top of your head, spreading throughout your body and radiating into your aura. If you wish, as the light enters your Crown chakra, you can visualise it refracting into the seven colours of the spectrum, with each colour being drawn into its designated chakra to balance and energise.

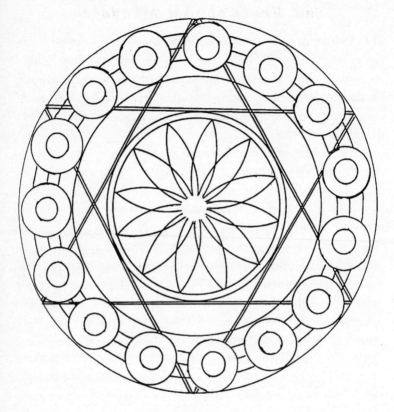

The Wheel of Life

The Wheel of Life Mandala

The Wheel of Life is sometimes known as the Wheel of Dharma and combines the symbolic meaning of the circle with movement. The wheel is sometimes used as the emblem for the whole cosmos, with its constant cycles of renewal and rebirth. It also represents the sun and the gods attributed to the sun.

Eastern philosophy teaches that we are all travelling around the Wheel of Life. With each life, we incarnate to the spoke that will give us the conditions needed for our growth and learning. Not until we have reached the state of realisation will we be free of these endless cycles.

The outer circles on this mandala represent our many lives on earth and contain the lessons learned and the progress made. At the centre lies the Flower of Life, whose petals radiate the light of the spiritual sun. The whole mandala is interlaced with the six-pointed star, pointing the way to perfection through the integration of all aspects of ourselves to a point of polarity.

As you work with this mandala, consider how this interpretation speaks to you. Do you feel comfortable with the idea of reincarnation? What are your thoughts on the Wheel of Life? When you have thought on these things, write down how you would interpret this mandala.

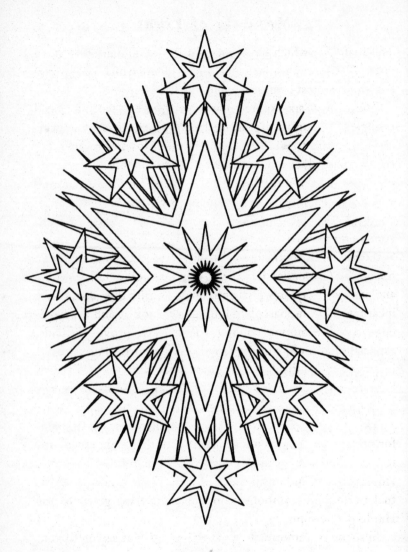

Mandala of Light

Mandala of Light

This mandala, which speaks of light, is not contained within a circle because that original light from which all things became manifest cannot be contained.

The central six-pointed star is formed by two interlaced triangles. The upward-pointing triangle is the masculine principle, relating to the fire element. The downward-pointing triangle is the feminine principle and is related to the element of water. The number six speaks of the harmony achieved when we are able to integrate our feminine and masculine energies. For many people, the concept of human beings containing both of these energies may be new. While looking at the mandala, think about this. If you have incarnated into a female body, ponder what role your masculine energy plays and consider ways in which you can work with this. If you have incarnated into a masculine body, then look at and acknowledge your feminine energy. This may prove difficult, especially for men, who are largely conditioned to think that it is 'unmanly' to display their emotional feelings. This is sad, because men working alongside their feminine energy heighten their sensitivity and artistic talents.

The number eight, found in the eight outer stars, stands for perfection. Yogic philosophy teaches that eight steps have to be observed in order to reach this perfected state. Hinduism and Buddhism speak of eight paths leading to spiritual perfection, symbolised in the eight arms given to the Hindu god Vishnu.

In silence, contemplate what this mandala is saying to you.

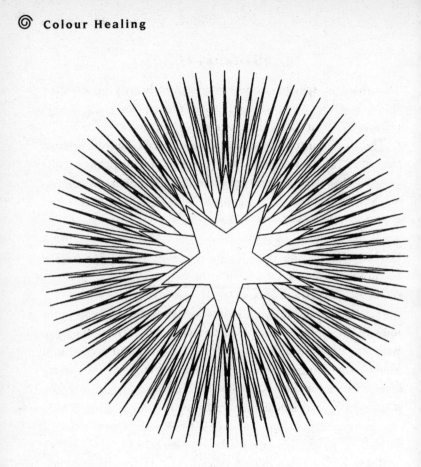

Starburst

Starburst

This mandala speaks of the radiance and beauty of our own inner light. As we work to create harmony and truth within ourselves so our inner light starts to glow more brightly.

The five-pointed star is symbolic of man, and the formation of the stars behind the central star represents the increased power and brilliance attained by our inner light as we walk along our chosen path. The rays that emanate from the stars form the protective coat of colour and light surrounding each of us. As we grow, the light becomes brighter and the colours more intense. When we fail to acknowledge our Divine Self, this light diminishes and the colours fade through lack of spiritual food.

As you contemplate this mandala, visualise your own inner light radiating from your Heart chakra and surrounding you with an auric coat of light and colour, beauty and protection. When colouring it, it is well worth doing several, using different combinations of colours. I found it amazing how the mandala changed when I changed its colours.

Switch on your light in all lives. Feel that you are the one life that shines in all creation.

Paramahansa Yogananda

9

Healing with Colour

Your whole body is light. Light is everywhere and all around you. Every moment God is making you anew, changing your atoms and cells and tissues. But your light is covered with darkness by the gross body. So shun your bad habits, be new, pure, perfect and divine.

Paramahansa Hariharananda Giri

The vibrational energies of colour are used for healing by colour practitioners in various ways.

Having worked as a colour practitioner for many years, I believe that the only person who can heal is the person to whom the disease belongs. For me, the physical body is the instrument that registers our mental, emotional and spiritual imbalances, stemming from either the conscious or unconscious mind. If only the physical ailment is worked with and not the cause, then physical symptoms will continue to manifest. One example is eczema, which is often treated allopathically with hydrocortisone cream. This indeed clears the eczema, but it may recur at a later stage, or the patient may contract asthma, as eczema and asthma have a very close relationship.

When using colour therapy we work with the physically manifested disease in order to keep the body in homeostasis, as well as dealing with the cause of the disease and any stagnated energy that may have accumulated in the etheric layer of the aura. Disease starts in the aura and if not treated at this level will eventually manifest as a physical disease. There are several ways of detecting stagnant etheric energy. In reflexology it is detected by the presence of pain or crystalline deposits found in the reflexes on the feet. In colour therapy it can be seen by people who have the gift of auric sight, or felt when the aura is scanned during a colour therapy treatment.

Of the two ways in which colour is reflected – as light (illuminatory) or as a pigment – light is the most powerful way of working with colour but it should only be used in therapy by a qualified practitioner. Contra-indications are associated with the use of certain illuminatory colours and if these are used in error more harm than good is done. The owner of a hair salon once contacted me. He had read that colour could relax a person as well as change their mood and had the idea of fitting a spare room in his salon with a set of rainbow-coloured lights. He then planned to ask his clients if they felt drawn to any specific colour; if they did he proposed to sit them in this room for half an hour, flooded with the colour of their choice. Not such a bright idea, in fact. If, for example, the client suffered heart problems, high blood pressure or asthma and they sat under red light for this length of time, the chances are that they would end up in hospital. If a person wishes to be treated with illuminatory colour, it is always advisable to seek a qualified colour practitioner. If you want to help yourself with colour, then work with pigment colour.

Treatments

It is advisable to explore the many ways that a person can be treated with colour before deciding which method you feel would be most beneficial. As discussed in Chapter 1, colour can be used in conjunction with a number of other therapies. It can also be administered through contact healing and the use of coloured lights. It is these techniques that I use when working with colour and I also combine it with reflexology treatment. Sometimes it is the patient who decides which particular method they wish to be treated with and sometimes it is myself.

When a patient attends for treatment, on their first visit it is usual to take down their details and medical history and, if they are suffering from a physical ailment, enquire whether or not they have sought medical advice. If they have not, I always suggest that they should. If a person is suffering abdominal pain, it could be appendicitis, which needs urgent medical treatment if peritonitis is to be avoided.

The patient is then encouraged to talk about themselves because this often helps them to find and work with the cause of the complaint. Following this, the appropriate treatment is given.

Contact Healing

If the form of treatment chosen uses colour with contact healing, the patient is asked to relax on a therapy couch. If they find it difficult to relax, the practitioner will help them by using one of the many relaxation techniques. Then, working from the head of the patient down to their feet, their aura is scanned for the presence of stagnated energy with the practitioner's hands. This is usually detected by the sensations of either cold, heat or pain. If a practitioner is able to see the aura, stagnated energy is observed as patches of grey mist lying over specific areas of the physical body. These areas of stagnation are then dispersed with colour, restoring the free flow of the patient's energy. The body is then worked down a second time, with the practitioner's hands making contact with the patient's body to channel the appropriate colours needed to work with any manifested disease and to help maintain the body in a state of homeostasis.

After treatment, the patient is encouraged to discuss any experiences or insights gained. They are then given instructions on how to work with the colour that will be most beneficial for them during the following week. This colour is known as the overall colour, because it treats the whole person and works with the cause of the disease. As a person changes as they work with themselves, the colour changes, which is why a colour is only worked with for one week. Treatments are normally at weekly intervals, which allows for any changes to be noted and a new colour given. There are several ways of finding the overall colour, such as kinesiology (muscle testing) and dowsing (working with a pendulum).

Coloured Light

Another treatment is the use of coloured light. To obtain the correct shade of a colour, stained-glass filters are used. When the overall colour has been determined, this and its complementary colour are projected through the colour therapy instrument to the patient in a darkened room for just under 20 minutes (see page 137). A darkened room is used because daylight dilutes colour. You can prove this for yourself by leaving a piece of material, dyed with a natural dye, in a sunlit room. After a while you will find that the colour fades.

For this form of treatment the patient is dressed in white

to allow the colour to be absorbed through the skin. If the colours are projected on to coloured clothes, the colour that the patient will receive will be a combination of the coloured light and the colour of their clothes. I also request that the patient keeps their eyes open throughout the treatment, so that the colour can penetrate their eyes. From research that has been carried out I personally feel that the projection of light and colour through the eyes has as great an effect as projecting it on to the body. When the treatment is finished, discussion is encouraged and instructions are given on how to work with these colours for self-help during the coming week until the next treatment. This advice follows every treatment.

Reflexology

A way in which I often use colour with patients is to combine it with a reflexology treatment. Over the years that I have been doing this I have seen some remarkable results. I have found it especially beneficial for people with very tender feet who find the pressure techniques of reflexology painful, for the terminally ill, and for conditions that have little response to reflexology alone. For me, combining colour with reflexology gives an added strength that works well with difficult ailments. It also causes no pain when projected on to painful reflexes. Students whom I have trained in this technique have also found these observations to be true.

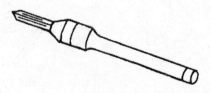

The reflexology torch

When combining colour with reflexology, one always starts the therapy session with a reflexology treatment, because this is diagnostic and also allows the location of stagnated energy, which is usually reflected as pain or crystalline formation in specific reflexes. The appropriate colour, with its complementary colour, is then administered to these reflexes through the reflexology crystal torch. An added benefit for the patient when working with this torch is again the absorption of the colours through their eyes. The treatment ends by balancing the chakras found on the spinal reflex on both feet and administering the overall colour through the feet with the reflexology colour instrument. This lasts for just under seven minutes. When working with very tense, nervous patients, I discovered that by putting blue followed by orange through the solar plexus reflex prior to the start of treatment the patient completely relaxes.

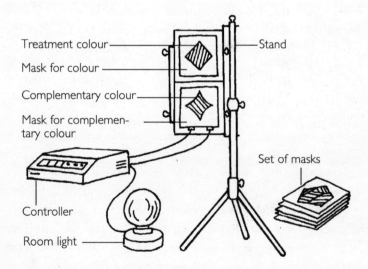

Treatment colour — Stand
Mask for colour
Complementary colour
Mask for complementary colour
Set of masks
Controller
Room light

The colour therapy instrument

Colour and Specific Illnesses

Many types of disease can be treated with colour therapy. Two problems that people frequently present are sinusitis and arthritis. Sinusitis seems to be on the increase, perhaps because of the level of pollution now present in the atmosphere or the large amounts of dairy produce being consumed. Dairy produce generates an overproduction of mucus in the body, and should be avoided by anyone suffering respiratory or sinus problems.

Mrs D., a patient whom had I treated some months before, attended with chronic sinusitis. She had suffered this for quite a long time, despite several courses of antibiotics prescribed by her doctor. When discussing her diet, it transpired that she ate a large amount of dairy produce in the form of cheese, butter and yoghurt. At the start of the treatment, I suggested she eliminated these from her diet for the next month. This she agreed to do while still attending weekly for colour treatment. Initially, her symptoms became worse, a normal occurrence as the body works to eliminate the excess mucus and any bacteria that may be present. At the end of the first month she reported an improvement in her condition and a greater sense of well-being. She continued to abstain from eating dairy produce and attended for four more treatments, at the end of which her sinuses were completely clear.

I usually treat arthritis with pure colour therapy. Diet again plays an important role in this condition. If the joints have become deformed, colour will not right them but colour therapy can alleviate the associated pain and prevent further bone deterioration. I have also discovered that deep-seated resentment can physically manifest as an arthritic condition.

Mrs E. attended complaining of arthritis in her knees, wrist and finger joints. She was taking anti-inflammatory drugs prescribed by her doctor, which she found helped her. It transpired that she had a very acidic diet, with lots of oranges, grapefruit, wine and meat. After we had discussed this, she agreed to see a nutritionist. Her life-style kept her indoors for most of the day and when she did manage to go outdoors she travelled by car because she found it painful to walk. Understanding the importance of the absorption of natural sunlight through the eyes for this condition, I recommended that she spent one hour each day outdoors. She agreed to try and do this, combining it with twice-weekly colour therapy treatments for the first month and then weekly treatments for a further two months. The first month of treatment showed a great improvement in her condition. The pain in her joints had lessened, enabling her to walk more easily and to have greater flexibility in her hands. After three months she was free from pain, had been taken off all drugs and was delighted with the way colour therapy had given her a new lease of life. She continued to come once every six weeks for what she called a 'top-up' treatment.

After a course of treatment for a specific illness, patients frequently continue to come once a month or once every six weeks in order to help maintain their state of well-being. This helps to release stress and tension and remove any stagnated energy present in the aura. In olden times patients would visit their acupuncturists on a regular basis to help keep their body in a state of balance. If the patient became ill, it was believed that the acupuncturist had not given good treatment so would have to pay the patient compensation.

I always tell my students that if they choose to work with other people they themselves will ultimately be 'tested'. I personally learned the truth in this saying when

I was admitted to hospital with a perforated appendix. After surgery I experienced a great deal of pain and the peristaltic action of my colon had stopped, a common occurrence with bowel surgery that prevents the patient from taking anything by mouth until the colon starts to work again. After three days of nothing happening, I decided to work on myself with the reflexology torch. I treated the reflexes on my hands relating to the small and large intestine and worked with colour over my abdomen. Four hours later the peristaltic action resumed, enabling me to start eating and then to return home – personal proof that the vibrational energies of colour really work in a healing capacity.

Some patients may not respond to colour and need to be referred to practitioners working with one of the other complementary therapies. I believe that the complexity of our individual nature makes each of us respond differently to the many therapies available.

If you decide that you would like to be treated with colour therapy, always attend a practitioner who has qualified through a recognised colour therapy school (see page 147). If you wish to use colour for first aid, to keep yourself healthy or to work with simple ailments then work with any of the techniques given in the previous chapters, but use only pigment colour. Please remember that if your symptoms persist medical advice must be sought.

Colour Chart for Simple Ailments

Condition	Pigment Colour	Methods of Application
headaches	medium blue	Visualise the colour flooding the whole of your face and head. Breathe the colour through the top of your head.

migraine	indigo	Use visualisation or colour breathing.
eye strain	indigo	Tie a blue silk or cotton scarf loosely over your eyes and look through it until your eyes feel rested.
stiff neck	medium blue	Tie an indigo silk or cotton scarf round your neck. Work with colour breathing.
sore throat	red	Tie a red silk or cotton scarf round your neck. Breathe this colour from the earth, into the part of your throat that feels sore.
asthma	medium blue	Breathe this colour into your lungs.
muscular strains	medium blue	Breathe in this colour and, as you exhale, visualise it being absorbed by the appropriate muscles.
general tension	medium blue	Visualise yourself lying in a field of cornflowers, imagining the blue displayed by the petals of the flowers being absorbed by every cell of your body. Wearing white, lie in a brightly lit room, under a length of blue silk or cotton material for 20 minutes.
indigestion	yellow	Breathe in yellow, visualising it flooding your stomach. Take note of your diet.
constipation	red	Visualise a ray of red light coming from the earth, into your feet and legs and into your colon. Take note of your diet.
depression	orange	Visualise an orange growing until it becomes the size of a room. Walk round the orange, find the door into the orange, enter and sit among the orange rays that penetrate the room you have just entered. Practise for at least 20 minutes each day.

pregnancy	blue	Visualise yourself surrounded by an orb of blue light that brings to you and your unborn child a wonderful sense of peace and relaxation. Wear blue clothes.
toxicity of the body	lime green	Visualise yourself sitting under a lime green waterfall that washes you inside and out. Take note of your diet.
arthritis	yellow and indigo	Fasten strips of yellow or indigo silk or cotton around the affected joints. Breathe yellow or indigo into these joints.
backache	medium blue	Breathe colour into your spine until it becomes completely encapsulated in this colour. If pain persists consult an osteopath or chiropractor.
sinusitis	red and green	Place both of your hands over your face and visualise a ray of red light coming through your feet, your body, into your hands and your sinuses. After five minutes, change the colour to green, bringing this colour horizontally into your Heart chakra, down your arms and into your hands.
common cold	orange	Lie under a piece of orange silk or cotton. Visualise yourself shrouded in an orange cloak. Drink plenty of fluids.
minor burns	turquoise	On top of a dry sterile dressing covering the burn, wrap a piece of turquoise silk or cotton material.
eczema	yellow and violet	Visualise the affected area bathed in a golden yellow. After five minutes, change the colour to violet.

Working With Terminally Ill Patients

During my years of working as a colour practitioner I have had some very positive and encouraging results with patients suffering terminal cancer as well as with those attending with minor ailments. When working with terminally ill patients in palliative care I realised that they were not necessarily going to be cured but that work with colour could give them a better quality of life and help them to die with dignity. Three patients in particular made a tremendous impression on me.

The first was Mr A., a terminally ill African who had lived in the United Kingdom for many years. I first met him at the day care centre that formed part of the palliative care unit. Medically all that could be done for him was pain control with morphine, which made him nauseous and caused constipation. In spite of this, he was always bright and cheerful, often singing spirituals to me while I treated him or giving me advice drawn from his own life experiences. During the three months that I treated Mr A. with a combination of reflexology and colour, his pain reduced and his nausea and constipation were alleviated, allowing for a reduction in his drugs. The last time I saw him, he had been admitted to a ward in the centre. As I left from giving him a treatment he laughed, thanked me for my help and told me that his maker had decided that it was now time for him to go home. He died a few days later.

Another patient I shall always remember was suffering motor neurone disease, a disorder of unknown origin where certain cells in the neurological system's motor nerves degenerate and die. I met Mr B. the day before he died and found him completely paralysed and having constant nursing care. I treated his feet with reflexology and colour and I shall always remember the look of appreciation and peace radiating from his eyes. His eyes were the only part of his body that he could move and this was how he made contact with people. I found this a wonderful example of the eyes being a mirror for the soul.

My third memorable experience in palliative care was with Mrs C., an elderly lady with terminal cancer whom I had been treating for several weeks. One particular week, when I entered her ward, the nurse stopped me to discuss their concern that the cancer was affecting Mrs C.'s brain, because she kept talking about the colours that she saw around people and objects. I thanked the nurse for this information then went to attend the patient. After starting the treatment, I asked Mrs C. if she could see colours around me. She nodded, so I asked her to tell me the colours she saw, which she did. I then asked her if she would like me to describe the colours I saw around her. As she nodded in agreement, tears came to her eyes and her face lit up, an experience which I will always remember. I have since questioned whether the morphine she was receiving had opened her auric sight. I still do not know the answer, but if morphine can do this to some people, it perturbs me to think that the medical profession has no understanding of this phenomenon and therefore relates it to a breakdown of one's mental faculties.

Since my time of working in palliative care I have had many cancer patients visit me for treatment. Some have been terminally ill and some in remission. With all these patients I have found that colour has had the power to alleviate some of the side effects of the drugs they were taking, creating for them a sense of peace and relaxation.

Finding a Colour Practitioner

If you have decided that you would like to be treated with colour therapy, you need to find a practitioner who is local to you and who has qualified through a school that is registered with either the Institute for Complementary Medicine (ICM) or the Complementary Medical Association (CMA). To register with either of these organisations, a practitioner must have trained with a school that they recognise as teaching to the required standard. The details of these associations can be found in the Useful Addresses section. Telephone or write to either or both of them asking for the name of a qualified practitioner in your area.

The number of visits that you will need will depend upon your state of health and how quickly you respond to treatment. It is usually recommended that you attend for a minimum of six visits, after which further visits may or may not be needed. If after the first or second treatment you decide that colour therapy is not right for you, then there should be no obligation for you make further appointments.

The cost of a treatment varies with each practitioner. It will also depend upon the part of a country where you are living. Practitioners in large towns usually charge more than those working in rural areas. An appointment at a health centre could also be more expensive than visiting someone who practises from home – a health centre has overheads to pay for.

If after your first visit you decide to continue treatment, it is important that you carry out any instructions on self-help that the therapist gives you. This aids the success of the treatment. I once treated a patient for chronic sinusitis who continued to eat large quantities of cheese. I advised that this should be eliminated from his diet, because it aggravated the problem by creating excess mucus. He failed to follow my advice with the result that his sinuses never completely cleared. I do feel that we are entering an age when we have to look at and learn to become responsible for ourselves. No longer can we expect others to take responsibility for us. Whether or not we work towards achieving this remains our choice.

Having read this book, if you decide to continue to work with the vibrational energies of colour, I hope that with practice you will also experience both its magic and power.

Useful Addresses

The Colour Bonds Association, 137 Hendon Lane, Finchley, London, N3 3PR. Tel/Fax: 0181 349 3299
(For information on colour therapy.)

Angelika Hochadel, International Mandel Institute, Dil-Mun, How Green Lane, Hever, Edenbridge, Kent, TN8 7PS.
(For information on colourpuncture.)

Complementary Medical Association (CMA), The Meridian, 142a Greenwich High Road, London, SE10 8NN. Tel/Fax: 0181 305 9571.

Institute for Complementary Medicine (ICM), Tavern Quay, Plough Way, Surrey Quays, SE16 1QZ. Tel: 0171 237 5165. Fax: 0171 237 5175

Light Information for Growth and Healing Trust (LIGHT), The Meridian Centre, 6 Larnach Close, Manor Park, Uckfield, East Sussex, TH22 1TH

Pauline Wills
The Oracle School of Colour

9 Wyndale Avenue, London, NW9 9PT. Tel/Fax: 0181 204 7672

(Please write to the above address for information on Practitioner Diploma Colour Courses and certified courses for integrating colour with reflexology.)

Further Reading

Allanach, Jack, *'Colour Me Healing' Colourpuncture: A New Medicine of Light*, Element, 1997

Alper, Dr Frank, *Exploring Atlantis*, 3 vols, Arizona Metaphysical Society, 1982

Birren, Faber, *Colour Psychology and Colour Therapy*, Citadel Press, 1950

Birren, Faber, *The Symbolism of Colour*, Citadel Press, 1989

Bonds, Lilian Verner, *Discover the Magic of Colour*, Optima, 1993

Cayce, Edgar, *Edgar Cayce on Atlantis*, Warner Books, 1968

Chaitow, Leon, *Relaxation and Meditation Techniques*, Thorsons, 1983

Clagett, Alice B. and Elandar Kirsten Meredith, *Yoga for Health and Healing from the teachings of Yogi Bhajan*, Alice B. Clagett, 1989

Cornell, Judith, *Mandala*, Quest Books, 1994

Goethe, Wolfgang von, *Theory of Colours*, MIT Press, 1970

Graham, Helen, *Healing with Colour*, Gill & Macmillan, 1996

Iyengar, Geeta S., *Yoga: A Gem for Women*, Allied Publishers Private Ltd, 1983

Krishnamurti, J., *Meditation*, Victor Gollancz Ltd, 1979

Le Shan, Lawrence, *How to Meditate*, Turnstone Press Ltd, 1974

Liberman, Jacob, *Light: Medicine of the Future*, Bear & Company, 1991

Ott, John N., *Health and Light*, Ariel Press, 1973

Shapiro, Eddie, *Inner Conscious Relaxation*, Element, 1990

Siegal, Bernie, *Peace, Love and Healing*, Rider, 1982

Silva, Mira and Mehta, Shyam, *Yoga – The Iyengar Way*, Dorling Kindersley, 1990

Wauters, Ambika, *Ambika's Guide to Healing and Wholeness: The Energetic Path to the Chakras and Colour*, Piatkus, 1993

Wills, Pauline, *Working with Colour*, Headway, 1997

Wills, Pauline, *Colour Therapy*, Element, 1993

Wills, Pauline, *Reflexology and Colour Therapy*, Element, 1992

Wills, Pauline, *The Reflexology Manual*, Headline, 1995

Wills, Pauline, *Visualization*, Hodder & Stoughton, 1996

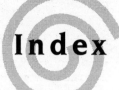

Index